feed your brain

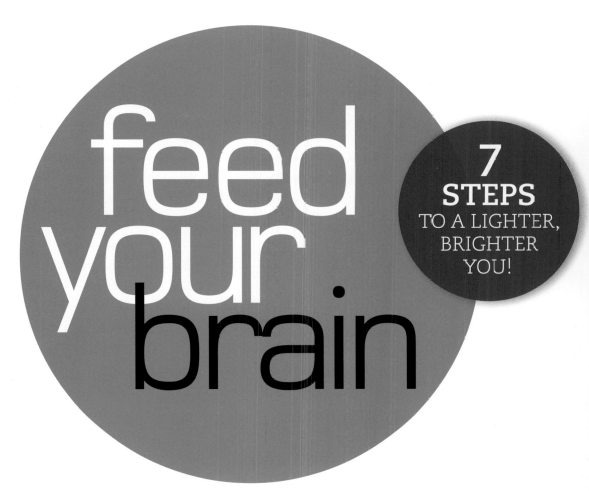

feed your brain

7 STEPS TO A LIGHTER, BRIGHTER YOU!

Includes Delicious Super-fast Recipes for Brain Health!

Delia McCabe

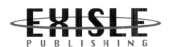

EXISLE
PUBLISHING

'I have had the great pleasure of hearing Delia McCabe speak on numerous occasions. Her extensive knowledge of the importance of feeding and nourishing the brain is not only inspiring, but has taught me so much about taking care of my own health. The information Delia shares is fuelled by her passion for healthy living and backed with solid research and facts. This book is a must read for anyone serious about taking care of their health!'
— *Jane Kerr*

'I'm the lowest weight I've been in twenty years and it's been so easy. I eat more and enjoy food more, and never count calories because I know that feeding my brain has helped my body become balanced! And I have no cravings! My brain is more focused and sharp, and my memory — which was always good — is now super sharp! I've got loads of energy again and even my sleep has improved. Every day I'm grateful for what Delia has taught me — it has transformed my life!'
— *Rae Antony*

'Delia's warm approach and clear communication skills have left guests mesmerized by her knowledge and ability to convert solid science into practical day-to-day advice. To see her healthy glow is a testament and a reflection of all the sayings — "Practice what you preach", "You are what you eat" — Delia "talks the talk and walks the walk"! It shows in every facet of her being. She is truly captivating! A highly intelligent, motivated woman, Delia's approach is simple: keep it real and apply knowledge in practical ways.'
— *Gregg Cave, Director and General Manager, Gaia Retreat and Spa*

'Learning from Delia is a true privilege. By applying what I learned from Delia my thinking is sharper, I am more focused, creative and enthusiastic, and my emotions are far more stable than ever before … it is TRULY amazing! For the first time in a long time, I have more control over how I feel — both physically and emotionally — and that, on its own, has been powerful as I live a super-busy life filled with continual challenges. '
— *Emily Gowor, author, speaker and entrepreneur*

'Watching my mother deteriorate after a diagnosis of Early Onset Dementia has motivated me to engage in healthier lifestyle choices as a means of prolonging onset (or better still) PREVENTING the development of Dementia in the future. I therefore felt privileged to be able to attend Delia's "Feed Your Brain" Workshop with an aim of nurturing my brain with more valuable (and scientifically driven) knowledge of brain health. Delia's focus is centred on proactive (preventable) actions rather than medically driven reactive solutions to chronic illness and disease. I am not a scientist, doctor, researcher or academic but I now feel like

I have the understanding and skills to further my knowledge of brain health and to use a holistic approach to preventative health that my family and I deserve.'
— *Jennifer Chastre*

'Delia's insight into what the brain needs to be fed — and what it's not getting anymore — explains the energy, weight, fatigue and memory woes that are plaguing the modern brain! Using a unique mix of psychology and neurology, Delia's genius around the stressed brain, sugar addictions, caffeine cravings and the ever-expanding muffin-top waistline, are unsurpassed! Delia provides hope, answers and solutions!'
— *Tanya Targett*

'I will always remember the first day I saw Delia speak. I felt she was speaking directly to me and I had quiet tears rolling down my face as I realized there may be help for the way I was feeling. I can't imagine what my health would be like now if I hadn't heard Delia speak and subsequently made the changes that she recommended. Delia summarizes complex science beautifully, and enabled me to implement changes at home which resulted in positive outcomes for us all, including my young son whose concentration and approach to school work has improved.'
— *K. Guthrie*

'Delia's extensive knowledge and research, which covers a range of complementary topics related to brain health — including fats and oils — is delivered with an authentic passion and personal humility that always makes her listeners want to learn more! Delia has mastered her delivery of scientific and sometimes complicated brain-focused content, so that it's easily understood and appreciated, and can be applied to our daily lives. Delia is one of the most trusted health advocates I know. I am always inspired to follow her guidance after watching her speak. Always!'
— *Jenni Madison, Coconut Magic*

'Delia has an insatiable knowledge of the relationship between food, mental health and exercise. Working as a dentist, in community health, I am aware of the complex issues surrounding mental health, but it has been Delia who has been an important reference for information about the impact of food on the mind and the body with the necessary focus on prevention.'
— *Dr Susan Stagg BDSC*

'Attending a talk given by Delia, I was completely amazed at her knowledge and insight. I'm not sure how she crammed so much amazing and thought-provoking information into that hour and a half — it must have taken years of research to condense and present the life-changing information Delia shared in such a concise and simple way! I wanted more at the end, as did everyone else in the audience!'
— *Robyn Rubenstein, psychologist*

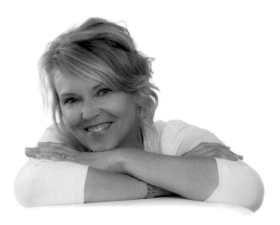

Delia McCabe has a Master's degree in Psychology but lost her enthusiasm for the 'talking cure' when she discovered that what you eat affects your brain function directly, and that until the brain is properly nourished, no amount of talking will get it working optimally. Instead, Delia decided to devote her time to extensively researching what the brain needs to function at its highest potential. The result is her unique seven-step plan that helps people to modify their eating habits without adding stress to their lives. She has seen time and again that the right diet can have a dramatic influence on one's memory, mood, ability to focus and stress levels. Apart from presenting workshops and conducting seminars, Delia is also presently completing her PhD, focused on the effects that specific nutrients have on female stress levels. Find out more about Delia and her work at www.lighterbrighteryou.life.

To my husband — my best friend — and my
children, who have patiently listened to my
excited explanations of why feeding the brain is so
important, and encouraged me to share this message
with others who want to feel the fabulous
benefits too.

First published 2016

Exisle Publishing Pty Ltd
'Moonrising', Narone Creek Road, Wollombi, NSW 2325, Australia
P.O. Box 60–490, Titirangi, Auckland 0642, New Zealand
www.exislepublishing.com

A CiP record for this book is available from the National Library of Australia.

ISBN 978 1 925335 11 8

Designed by Big Cat Design

Food styling and photography by Vanessa Russell from Raspberry Creative, with
the exception of the photograph on page 243 (courtesy of Shutterstock).

Illustrations courtesy of Luke McManus and Mark Thacker from references
supplied by the author, with the exception of the brain illustration on the cover
and the illustrations on pages ix, 16, 26, 136, 166, 170, 176, 182, 192, 199, 203,
216, 226 and 238 (courtesy of Shutterstock).

Typeset in Minion Pro 11.45 / 17.5pt
Printed in China

This book uses paper sourced under ISO 14001 guidelines from well-managed
forests and other controlled sources.

10 9 8 7 6 5 4 3 2 1

Photographic note
All food photographs were shot using an iPhone 6.

Disclaimer
This book is a general guide only and should never be a substitute for the skill,
knowledge and experience of a qualified medical professional dealing with the
facts, circumstances and symptoms of a particular case. The nutritional, medical
and health information presented in this book is based on the research, training and professional experience of the author, and is true and complete to the
best of their knowledge. However, this book is intended only as an informa-
tive guide; it is not intended to replace or countermand the advice given by the
reader's personal physician. Because each person and situation is unique, the
author and the publisher urge the reader to check with a qualified healthcare
professional before using any procedure where there is a question as to its
appropriateness. The author, publisher and their distributors are not responsible
for any adverse effects or consequences resulting from the use of the information in this book. It is the responsibility of the reader to consult a physician or
other qualified healthcare professional regarding their personal care. This book
contains references to products that may not be available everywhere. The intent
of the information provided is to be helpful; however, there is no guarantee of
results associated with the information provided.

contents

Preface

'If I could just follow one thought about a task that needs doing, and get that task done, I'd be fine,' Mary* confided in me. She had been under a lot of stress lately and was battling to complete tasks efficiently. 'It's as if I start a task and another thought gets in the way, and then I start that task and another jumps out at me. I really don't know what to do about it!' She mentioned that if she carried on like this her family would think she was losing her mind. I could see she was anxious and distressed, scared that her thoughts were too scattered for her to be able to function effectively.

'I just can't seem to think straight anymore,' Tom* said to me. He had explained that he was feeling quite down, and was lacking energy. He had tried a detox diet and it had only left him feeling worse. He told me that he felt he was losing his edge. 'The younger guys in the office are gaining on me, and if I don't get my act together, I'm sure I'll end up losing my job!' As he shakily reached for another swallow of his large cup of coffee, I knew he was feeling pretty desperate.

'Ever since I came down with the flu, I've felt really depressed. Although I'm well now, I just can't seem to shake this blue feeling. I was already feeling overwhelmed at work, and with my teenage sons, but now I feel much worse. I always used to have so much energy and could just keep going, but that's also changed. And I'm putting on weight!' Kathy* spoke quickly, and laughed, trying to make light of how she felt, and I could see that she was feeling guilty about what she saw as complaining.

More alarmingly, a young teenage girl, overhearing my discussion with a family member, said that she also needed some 'brain food'! She said she felt as if her memory was

1

failing her and worried about whether it was going to get worse. She thought she was too young to be experiencing memory challenges, but felt that her memory had been better when she was younger.

When I asked each of these people whether they thought food could help them feel better, they looked at me in astonishment. 'How can food help me think sharper?' 'Keep my thoughts in order?' 'And not be depressed?', they all asked individually. Countless others have replied in a similar way to the same question.

Fortunately for them (and for you), I've been thinking about and researching those exact questions for many years, and wrote this book to show you how food can help your brain (and the rest of you) stay happy, healthy and young for as long as possible. You see, this book will show you that when you feed your brain, you can change your life.

These people's challenges are examples of the many experiences I regularly hear about. Unfortunately, many people also contact me online and discuss their emotional distress with me, citing anxiety and depression as the two biggest burdens that they bear, day in and day out. They fear they are alone with these challenges, not realizing that there are millions of people who feel the same way, and who are suffering real distress because they can't find relief in anything but a tablet, which is short-lived anyway, and which comes with horrid side effects.

When you give your brain the nutrients it needs to function optimally, you naturally improve your mood, your weight stabilizes and you start losing weight if you need to. Your brain works more efficiently, improving learning potential, focus and memory and you become lighter in mood and weight, and brighter in outlook and cognitive capacity. Due to the brain being the 'greediest' organ in the body, when it is satisfied it sets off a wonderful 'domino effect' or cascade of improved health on every level.

* Names have been changed to protect the individuals' identity.

Introduction

A real interest in and fascination with the brain has been growing rapidly in recent decades, parallel to the astonishing advances science has made in looking inside our living brains. 'Seeing' inside a living brain gives us a glimpse of this magnificent organ in action. We now understand that, like the body, the brain is made up of flesh and blood and can be influenced by the same things that affect our body.

Using sophisticated technology, we can now see where activity is taking place in the brain and how much energy is being used in those specific areas. We can even get a very good idea of the health of the brain by using specific imaging techniques that tell us where damage has occurred and where tumours are hiding.

Without these forms of technology, the brain would have remained a mystery to us, just as it was up until the early twentieth century. Prior to these advancements, the only way people could study the brain was to look at it after death had arrived.

The first technique used in 1918 to investigate the brain was dangerous and painful. A technique called pneumoencephalography, pioneered by American neurosurgeon Dr Walter Dandy, drained cerebrospinal fluid (CSF) from around the brain and replaced it with air, enabling the subsequent change in the density of the brain relative to its surroundings to provide clear x-ray images of the organ. This was obviously a risky undertaking, with bleeding and infection as possible outcomes, but it was also dangerous because it increased the pressure inside the brain and was intensely painful! However, it allowed us to see both the surface of the brain and its ventricles, which was a huge breakthrough. The development of painless scanning techniques took us out of the dark ages and into a new world of possibilities, although it was only in 1977 that we actually got to see what the brain had been hiding with the development of human magnetic resonance imaging (MRI). Since then, the technology that is allowing us to investigate the last frontier of human anatomy has been growing in leaps and bounds. We can now produce images of neural pathways using diffusion tensor imaging (DTI), which shows us where connections between neurons exist and how they communicate with each other. Having gained knowledge of the actual brain structures, this new technology allows us to look at how neurons function and, ultimately, how the billions of neurons within the magnificent brain work together so beautifully.

Although we have uncovered many of its mysteries to date, there is still so much more to discover about the brain. Apart from being an organ made of flesh and blood, and being such a fascinating area of science to investigate, the brain has a deeper, more personal meaning to us. It is the seat of our entire being: it underpins how we love, how we hate, how we grieve and the way we think, plan, imagine, consider, dream and learn. It also co-ordinates our emotions and desires with our body so we laugh, feel fear or experience anticipation. How we move and play is according to its directives and the interactions that take place within its soft and spongy universe.

The brain itself is a physical organ held in place by the hard bones of our skull, but what is more fascinating is the mind that it holds within — something which is unique to each of us. Without the brain, there would be no mind and there would be no you! Your mind is forever changing and growing as you add to your experiences of life, so it is an evolving and deeply personal part of you.

There is nothing more central to a fulfilling life than an optimally functioning brain. If you want to preserve your mind and who you are in essence, you have to focus on pre-serving your brain. Because thinking is a pattern of cellular activity that occurs across a vast network of cells, chemicals, membranes and molecules, it is possible to influence the brain's functioning in the same way that we influence our body's functioning.

With a worldwide ageing population and cases of dementia, as well as severe depression and anxiety, alarmingly on the rise, the need to look after your brain optimally has never been more important. Cases of attention deficit hyperactivity disorder (ADHD), Asperger's disorder, autism and severely challenging learning disorders are also on the rise among our youth.

Data collected from 187 countries, reported in the 2010 Global Burden of Diseases, Injuries and Risk Factors Study, highlighted that mental disorders and substance abuse combined were the leading cause of non-fatal illness, contributing to nearly 23 per cent of the total global disease burden. Another alarming statistic is that 11 per cent of the US population over the age of twelve is using antidepressant medication. Americans alone spent more than US$11 billion on antidepressants in 2010.

Almost half of the Australian population will experience a mental illness in their lifetime and between 2008 and 2009, AU$743 million was spent on mental health medications in this country. The cost of mental illness in the UK is £77 billion, greater than heart disease and cancer combined. These are alarming figures, even more so when you consider that it is not just middle-aged patients who are visiting their doctor to get prescriptions filled for mind-altering medications.

Millions of children are also being diagnosed with mental health challenges too, often starting with ADHD medication and then moving on to other varieties of potent pharmaceuticals. In fact, there is startling research that reveals that people who are treated for an initial mental illness episode are significantly more susceptible to increased episodes of more severe mental challenges. So the child treated for ADHD with Ritalin is more likely to experience more severe psychological distress over time than the child who was not treated with any type of medication at all. Millions of children are also being treated with antidepressants, something that was quite unheard of a few decades ago.

It would be a very naïve and simplistic explanation to suggest that the dramatic change in diet over the past few decades is the only reason people are suffering from increased mental health challenges. There are, of course, a multitude of converging reasons for a mental health problem to occur. The environment, which includes the toxins we are exposed to, as well as the stress that we experience, and our genetic predisposition, all influence mental health. However, the brain, being made from the same flesh and blood as the rest of the body, requires specific nutrients to operate optimally. It will become less capable of managing effectively in the overwhelming world we find ourselves in today if it is not nourished properly. This book is an explanation of the basic nutritional principles (and some extra non-nutritional ones) the brain needs to operate optimally. These principles should form the foundation of your wellbeing so you can cope more efficiently and even thrive in the complex world we live in today. You will learn how to create a lighter, brighter you by supplying your brain with what it needs for optimum functioning.

Your brain and food

Fortunately, there is scientific proof to support the fact that what you eat can and does directly influence your mood, behaviour, concentration, learning and memory. You can literally feed your brain to be happy or sad and help it to learn and remember things much more efficiently, simply by changing the type of foods you eat.

Every meal and snack you consume, or feed your family, is either supporting healthy brain function or undermining it. Thankfully, you do not need to swallow horrid concoctions or eat boring, bland food to support your brain's glowing health. When you keep in mind that the best food is unprocessed and natural, and you learn how to make it tasty and enticing with the right fats, herbs and spices, you will enjoy supporting your brain, which is also your hungriest organ. And you will naturally find yourself feeling lighter and brighter!

My academic background is in psychology, not nutrition. But after twenty years of research into how nutrition influences brain function, I've had to learn a lot about food and what it does for the brain.

I came to study food and how it influences brain function when I realized that being a talking therapist was not for me. In fact, I felt that I would be dishonest if I tried to talk someone 'better', especially as I'd already discovered that many people who feel bad psychologically eat poorly. It happened like this.

While completing my Master of Psychology degree, I was working with a group of very smart adolescents. Although they were all capable of achieving well at school, many were, in fact, doing very poorly. I had a bit of extra space on one of the questionnaires I'd asked them to complete, so I threw in a few questions about what their favourite foods were. All the adolescents who were battling at school loved junk food, whereas the control group, the group who were smart and doing well, didn't! When I discovered this, I made a decision to investigate why this should be the case and in so doing, made the decision that being a therapist wasn't going to work for me. So you could call me a disillusioned or cynical would-be psychologist!

Many years later I have found that most people do not associate what they eat with how their brain is functioning. If they are forgetful, or moody, or battling to learn something new, they often look for other reasons to explain why they are feeling that way. What they eat never seems to come up for discussion. In addition, they reach for another coffee, or a chocolate bar, hoping that the energy-high won't wear off as quickly as it did the last time.

So I decided to write a book to explain why certain foods are great for maintaining great mental health, stable moods, improved focus and concentration, as well as enhanced memory capacity. Feeding your brain what it needs is a natural way to feel happier and enjoy more stable moods. As a result, you will also lose weight and improve your cognitive ability — leading to a lighter and brighter you!

If you know what various nutrients do in your brain and why they are critically important for optimal brain function, you'll be better equipped to choose your foods appropriately. Food is actually information and it can lead to optimal brain functioning, or dysfunction. We live in a super sophisticated and complex world. Navigating this world and thriving within its complexity produces levels of stress that we have not encountered as a species before. A stressed brain uses up more nutrients than a calm, relaxed brain, and also produces many more damaging cells called free radicals. This is one of the primary reasons why eating the right kinds of foods to support brain health is a real priority today, if you want to keep your cognitive edge. As an added bonus, there are no negative side effects from feeding your brain optimally! Extra energy, glowing skin, weight loss and improved moods are great side effects and no one is ever going to complain about that!

Fortunately, my psychology training did come in handy at various points during this journey of discovery, especially in how I share this knowledge because I understand why most people don't make positive changes in their life. Too much information presented too quickly and in too much detail may lead to interest initially, especially if it offers long-term solutions to unpleasant problems; however, eventually it will be discarded because no one can make a lot of changes in a short time. New habits take time to become part of a person's daily routine because new neural pathways have to be established and this doesn't happen overnight.

This book is divided into seven chapters. Each chapter contains information about a different topic, directly related to brain function. The aim is to incorporate each of the seven steps into your life so that your brain becomes well nourished and can serve you in the best way possible. Each chapter is made up of small sections, each with a heading that relates to what the section is about. If you simply want to scan the headings and read what is interesting to you first, then go ahead. If you want more in-depth knowledge, then you should read each chapter in its entirety, as well as the information boxes. At the end of each chapter I have provided you with an action plan to give you an idea of how to implement that chapter's information into your life.

Although the book starts with a 'non-food' chapter, it is an introduction into how you can start nourishing your brain in ways that you may not have considered before. From Chapter 2 onwards, the discussion on the role of food in brain health will unfold, revealing how you can transform your life by feeding your brain. In addition, I've provided the basic nutritional science of what your brain likes and needs, what it doesn't like and what damages it. If you want to find out more about the research, the reference list at the end of the book is a good place to start.

Some important brain facts

Concentration, focus, memory and mood all occur across an enormous network of sophisticated, interconnecting brain cells, called neurons. Each of these specialized cells depends on an optimal supply of nutrients from the food we eat, in order to work smoothly and efficiently. Without the right nutrients your brain is incapable of working effectively. In addition, simply adding a multi-nutrient, like a vitamin tablet or a green drink, to a poor diet isn't going to do the trick either.

Let's have a look at a few of the wondrous things most people don't know about the brain:

- The brain weighs between 1.3 to 1.4 kg (2.9 to 3.1 lbs) and is only about 2 per cent of your body weight.

- It uses 25 per cent of the oxygen that you breathe, which is every fourth breath, to put it into context.

- It uses up to half of the glucose that your body produces from carbohydrates for its energy requirements.

- Each unit of brain tissue needs 22 times the amount of metabolic energy compared to the same amount of muscle tissue.

- The brain uses 20 per cent of the heart's output of blood (i.e. 25 times more blood than the equivalent weight of resting tissue).

- One-fifth of the heart's activity is in the service of the brain.

- At any given moment in time, your brain is receiving and processing approximately 100 million pieces of information.

- You will lose consciousness in about 8 to 10 seconds, if the blood supply to your brain is cut off.

- There are anywhere from 1000 to 10,000 synapses (links between brain cells) for each neuron.

- There are 160,000 kilometres (100,000 miles) of blood vessels in the brain — the distance it would take you to go around the world approximately four times.

- In response to mental activity, the brain continues to grow new neurons.

- Information can travel between neurons as slowly as 0.5 metres (1.6 feet) per second, or as fast as 120 metres (390 feet) per second, which is about 430 kilometres (268 miles) per hour.

- It is a myth that humans only use 10 per cent of their brain. All the parts of the brain are used; however, some people use their brains more efficiently than others.

- Every time you blink (20,000 times per day) the brain steps in and keeps the world illuminated for your neurons so that everything doesn't go black.

Three concepts to grasp about brain function

We can break down the approach to brain function into three very broad concepts. The first area assesses what the actual hardware of the brain needs to perform optimally. So, looking at the cells (neurons) and their supporting cells (the glia) in specific areas of the brain, as well as the various specialized chemicals and electrical impulses that move around in the brain, we get a good idea of what they all require to perform their duties effectively. The second area involves examining the feelings or emotions that you experience, such as love, frustration, devotion, irritability and compassion. Memory, learning and focus also fall into this domain, although they are not feelings but cognitive states of mind and mental capacities. It's a private and personal area. No one can see these feelings or mental states, yet they are real. The aim is to increase the amount of feelings that you enjoy experiencing, and improve cognitive functioning in a simple and direct way by feeding your brain optimally. The third area is the result of these two areas interacting. The external manifestation of what is going on inside your head is your behaviour, which can include your facial expressions, your actions and movements, and the words you utter. When something goes wrong in the flesh of your brain, the hardware, your emotions and cognitive capacity will be influenced, and then as a consequence, your behaviour. This is why it's easier to first work on what is going wrong in your brain before we try to change your feelings and behaviour. This is why the 'talking cure' can be very frustrating for both the therapist and the client when the client's brain is malnourished.

Lifestyle choices and cognitive wellbeing

Lifestyle choices will influence both physical wellbeing and mental health. Research shows this clearly today. Research also shows clearly that cognitive decline isn't inevitable with age and that there are, in fact, specific things you can do and others you can avoid that may prevent your cognitive decline. And having genes that may predispose you to poor mental health is not your destiny. After all, only one-third of the way you age is determined by your genetic make-up, the other two-thirds are under your control.

How the brain changes due to experience and learning is a physical occurrence in the brain's 'hardware', with psychological and behavioural results. The technical name for this ability is 'neuroplasticity'. The brain's grey matter is made up of millions of neurons which can stay robust or shrink in size, and the connections between these neurons can be strengthened or weakened, or new ones can be created. This is where new skills and abilities are first created, and then we can act them out because our brain has a new neural pathway. These changes on the physical terrain of the brain give new instructions to the body, which manifest as new abilities and skills. When you forget someone's name or why you walked into a room, this is a sign of weakening connections to that memory. So you can focus on keeping the connections strong and robust and forging new ones, or you can allow your brain to shrink and therefore become diminished as a person in the process. If you have read this far, you aren't going to let that happen.

In one research study led by Dr Sabia, over 5000 men and women were followed for a period of seventeen years, with the aim of looking at what their lifestyles were like and how they aged cognitively. The results were fascinating and showed how much control we have over how our brain ages, as the number of unhealthy behaviours (smoking, low physical activity, low fresh produce consumption), and the duration of these behaviours were associated with cognitive decline in later life.

Another recent study led by Dr Tasnime Akbaraly examined the impact of diet on overall health in older people and found that a high intake of fried and sweet foods, as well as processed foods, red meat, refined grains and high-fat dairy products led to less healthy outcomes than a diet focused on whole foods, such as wholegrains, polyunsaturated fats, nuts and fruit and vegetables. In addition, they found that mental and cognitive function was influenced negatively by poor food choices. These studies are robust in that they examine the person and their food choices over a long period of time.

So, the current research into the brain indicates very clearly that cognitive decline is not inevitable with ageing. We can take very practical and simple steps to maintain our cognitive health throughout our lives due to neuroplasticity and the brain's ability to create new pathways. As individuals, we have to take responsibility for our own cognitive health, in an ever-ageing population.

Another large research study led by Dr Martin Loef looked at factors that led to good health. They summed up their findings and declared that there are five primary areas that we need to keep in mind when we look at how we feel, how we are ageing and what our health status is:

1. never smoking
2. having a body mass index (BMI) lower than 30
3. being physically active for 3.5 hours per week
4. following healthy dietary guidelines, such as a high intake of fruits and vegetables, wholegrain bread and low meat consumption, and
5. consuming a moderate amount of alcohol.

A magic potion ... ?

Although there are many marketing strategies advising which specific nutrient or compound will ensure a healthy brain that doesn't age, these are simply marketing strategies to sell you the item. This is not to say there aren't particular supplements that can help you maintain your brain, it's just that this is not the only solution to a well-maintained brain.

Secondly, all the research points to prevention being better than cure. This is not a new refrain. If you want a brain that's going to work well into old age, you need to start thinking about its welfare before you suffer from any mental complaint. It's much harder to get yourself well than it is to keep yourself well. If you keep these two points in mind, this book will be valuable for you. If you want to throw your money at the latest 'brain' fad, you are welcome to do so. But, you will find yourself back here, reading these words, when the 'magic bullet' didn't deliver all it promised.

Why is your diet the simplest way to influence your brain?

We eat a number of times every day. While eating provides nourishment to fuel our brain and body, it is also a great source of pleasure and provides an opportunity to interact with our loved ones and friends. Using food to keep your brain working well, once you know which are the best brain-supportive foods, is the simplest way to stay sharp. Because nutrients go to work very quickly to either support great mental function or to undermine it, you can quickly see a cognitive 'result' after eating. Although coffee can give you a very quick energy 'hit', a snack that provides good fats, protein and unrefined carbohydrates, like a handful of almonds or goji berries or sun-dried tomatoes, will provide an energy boost that won't drop off quickly because it helps keep blood glucose levels stable.

Eating well to support your brain is also really simple once you know how. After all, it's a lot simpler than following complex computer games, doing Sudoku and crossword puzzles, and learning a new language, although these activities also improve cognitive function. But you can't really do them as regularly as eating!

Maybe you're curious about how food can improve your brain? The simple answer is that food can help to:

- improve your clarity of mind

- increase your speed of thinking or cognitive processing

- enhance your ability to pay attention

- lengthen the amount of time you can concentrate for

- improve your memory and learning capacity, and

- improve and sustain your positive mood.

Today we often eat more because of the pleasure of eating, rather than because we are driven from an internal desire to satisfy true hunger. The natural environment that surrounded us during early human existence didn't always provide us with a reliable and regular food supply. We had to adjust to this variability in food supply, and our adaptive mechanisms for handling this situation involved our consumption of large quantities of foods when it was available, enabling temporary fat storage, and coping with meagre supplies when that was the situation.

We developed flexibility in relation to our appetite and satiety mechanisms. An obese person would have been at a disadvantage when having to flee a predator, and a very thin person with no energy reserves would have been in a similarly disadvantaged position.

However, we have vast quantities of food at our disposal today, and it may be that some people react to this constant supply in a way that would resemble their ancestors' response — they 'stock' up for times of famine. This is one of the many reasons why people are getting more and more overweight — it's very hard to have self-restraint in a society where there is so much delicious food available 24/7. This has, unfortunately, led to a new phenomenon called 'affluent malnutrition' or the undernourishment of essential nutrients. Today, people are eating food that is high in energy value or calories, but very low in nutrients. In the past, we suffered from diseases that were often caused from a lack of food, such as a lack of citrus foods causing scurvy. Today, in the western world, we have access to too much food, and too many of the wrong ones, which are causing many diseases. Malnutrition is caused through a lack of the correct nutrients, an imbalance of nutrients, or an excess of the wrong kind of nutrients.

The other interesting aspect to this process of eating is that we have an innate preference for foods that have sweet, salty or fatty tastes. This ensured that we searched for and consumed a range of foods, which would improve our chances of getting a variety of necessary nutrients. We have an evolutionary desire for sweetness, due to the ability of dense carbohydrates to give us a quick energy boost — which is very helpful when you're starving, but not much good when you live in the land of refined, processed and sugar-laden carbohydrates, as we do now.

Our internal mechanisms to control appetite and satiation haven't evolved to take this into account. It is therefore very easy to overeat, usually on the very foods that do not sustain optimal cognitive function.

Choices

This book is about choices supported by science: choices for people who may believe that they have no control over how their brain works and ages; choices for people who fear that their genes are their destiny and that the statistics of mental illness, brain disease and disability are inevitable for them. When you focus on ill health and disease, you will see nothing but hopelessness and despair. When you focus on all the wonderful new research that we have at our disposal, you will see that you have choices and will understand that statistics are not destiny, and that knowledge gives you power.

Combining the right choices from each of the chapters, coupled with my advice, will enable you to nourish your brain and in so doing become lighter and brighter naturally. Following these steps is not complicated and doesn't require a huge financial investment. By simply making different choices, you can experience profound change, both mentally and physically.

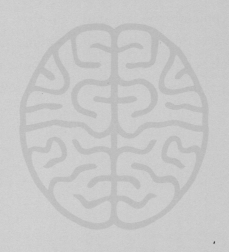

part 1

brain basics

CHAPTER 1

Sweat, sleep, sex and stress — what they mean to your brain

Although sweating more, improving sleep, making great sex a priority and reducing stress are not food-related ways to improve brain function, they are all activities that nourish the brain. Research into these four activities is growing, especially on why we should be doing more of the first three and getting rid of the last one.

The aims of this chapter are to give you a very clear explanation of why getting your body and brain to sweat is good for your thinking processes, as well as for mood and memory. It will also explain the importance of sex and sleep, what sleep does to your brain and why stress is damaging to your brain.

Sweating for your brain

There is a vast array of research indicating that exercise is good for you, with most studies focusing on heart health. But what is also known is that what's good for your heart is also good for your brain. Why? The first artery, the carotid artery, which comes out of the heart carrying freshly oxygenated blood, goes to the brain. This means that your brain immediately gets the first flush of fresh oxygen and nutrients to sustain its health when you exercise. Exercise also increases the growth of specific neuronal cells, called astrocytes, which support neurons in their highly specialized activities, and less inflammation occurs in the brain due to this increased blood flow In addition, specific neurotransmitters are increased after exercising, which will give you a feeling of being calm, yet focused and less impulsive. You also reduce the risk of getting Type 2 diabetes when you exercise regularly, a risk factor for developing anxiety, depression and Alzheimer's disease.

Interestingly, exercise that increases your heart rate also increases your ability to pay attention, which in turn increases the chances of you being able to recall what you are learning. Your learning ability is enhanced immediately after exercising, so that what you learn will be retained and can be retrieved later on. There are some progressive schools that are capitalizing on this phenomenon to ensure that their students' brains are receptive to what they learn just after an aerobic workout.

Other positive benefits of exercise include the possible potential to restore some of the cognitive functions that have been lost due to normal ageing; and to enhance some cognitive functions in the brain, especially in the hippocampus (one of the main memory centres in the brain) and in the frontal cortex (the management centre that oversees decision making, rational thinking and long-term thought processes). Exercise also helps your brain to produce energy more efficiently, which means that it's easier for it to work well.

Fertilizer for your brain

The next reason why exercise benefits your brain starts deep within your muscles. Chemicals are sent from your working muscles into your bloodstream, which then cross the blood–brain barrier into your brain. These chemicals then start increasing the production of another very important chemical called brain-derived neurotrophic factor, or BDNF, which acts like fertilizer for your neurons, encouraging them to stay healthy and keep growing, even helping to grow new neurons.

When you exercise regularly, your brain builds up reserves of BDNF and your neurons start to branch out, joining together and forming new connections. This is what underlies new learning — every new connection made between your neurons is a sign of a new skill or fact or name that you have learnt, and that you are putting into storage for future use. So, brains with more BDNF have a greater capacity for learning new things.

Now, the opposite holds true too — a brain that has no or very low supplies of BDNF is a brain that switches off to new knowledge, and has trouble recalling already stored information. As we age, our levels of BDNF fall, but researchers have found that exercise induces their production and can therefore help to maintain levels.

But that's not the whole story because science has revealed that BDNF is also responsible for the growth of new neurons called neurogenesis, which was believed to be impossible up until a few years ago. When researchers looked at where these new neurons were growing, they discovered that it was primarily in the hippocampus, the area of your brain responsible for learning and memory. When you can't match a face to a name, this is the area of your brain that is battling to retrieve the information.

The good news is that exercise can help the BDNF to restore those neurons to a healthier state, and also reverse some of the damage that has already occurred. There is even more good news. Your frontal lobes, which oversee and dictate decision making and planning, as well as pattern detection and self-discipline, can get bigger if you exercise regularly. Having optimally functioning frontal lobes increases your enjoyment of life because you will make better decisions, be more goal-orientated and enjoy a better, more positive outlook on life. You will naturally feel 'brighter' about your life because your goals, aspirations and capabilities will be clearer.

The blood–brain barrier

The blood–brain barrier is a specialized system of sophisticated cells that form a barrier against toxic and harmful compounds entering the brain. The brain receives the same blood that flows through the body, so this system works to keep out compounds that could harm sensitive brain tissue. Some parts of the brain never develop a barrier at all, such as the hypothalamus and the pineal gland, both critically important for normal brain (and body) function. The cells in the blood–brain barrier can be compromised in their protective function during certain infectious states, from head injury and degenerative conditions. Certain viral and bacterial infections of the brain and spinal cord will also cause barrier ineffectiveness, as will hypertension and exposure to some heavy metals such as tin and lead. An elevated core body temperature, which occurs during heat stroke, can do the same thing, as can severe hypoglycaemia (low blood sugar). Ageing is also thought to lead to less effective barrier protection, making the ageing brain especially vulnerable to toxins that can cause harm. In addition, this barrier becomes temporarily ineffective or less effective during strokes (even small or 'silent' ones), which results in brain swelling.

Exercise and mitochondria

In Chapter 6 you will learn about carbohydrates and how your cells produce energy in tiny little factories called mitochondria. Without these tiny structures, our cells would be unable to produce the energy we need to function. Currently, they are being studied in great detail because they may hold the key to managing disease and ageing, including brain ageing.

One of the most interesting findings is that when you do aerobic exercise, you actually increase the number of mitochondria present in your muscle cells by 40 to 50 per cent in about six weeks. The outcome of this is less fatigue, less exertion required when exercising and greater endurance. This is because your mitochondria are burning fat more efficiently, rather than carbohydrate, for energy.

To get this benefit you need to walk briskly, cycle, swim, run or do other heart rate-raising exercises for at least 15 to 20 minutes a day, three to four times a week. To maintain this new level of increased mitochondria, you will have to keep exercising regularly.

As you age, your mitochondria work less efficiently, which is why the focus is on keeping them healthy, and exercise is another way of doing this very effectively. It looks as if exercise helps to slow down the mitochondria ageing process. This phenomenon is not limited to the muscles of the body — the mitochondria in the brain, specifically in the hippocampus, become more efficient at producing energy and this in turn also influences the ability of neurons to grow, adapt and change.

Sweat and toxins

Many of the toxins that are present in our foods and the environment find their way into our fat cells and the membranes of our cells and stay there. Unfortunately, they also find their way into our very fatty brains. The fastest and most efficient way to get rid of these toxins is to sweat them out — being fat-soluble they work their way out of our fatty pores through perspiration.

As Chapter 7 will reveal, consuming the right fats is an integral part of brain health, and fortunately the bad fats get replaced with the good ones when you provide them. So, sweating through exercise allows the body to get rid of the bad fats, where the toxins are lodged, and replace them with the good ones that you will start eating. This process will occur naturally in your brain too, when you start consuming the right fats.

Stimulate your senses

One of the reasons we lose cognitive ability as we get older is because our senses are unable to operate at their peak level. This means our eyes, ears and skin are not as sensitive as they were in our youth and so we perceive our environment and those we interact with, with less sensitivity. This leads us to respond in ways that are not conducive to laying down memory traces, and being unable to recall what we have experienced. It also impacts our ability to learn. As a result, we become less attentive, more forgetful and easily distracted. Having your eyes and ears tested is the first step to ensuring that your brain is getting good information to store and use.

Another way to ensure the brain continues to operate efficiently is to be busy and involved in activities during normal life, such as reading, travelling, playing card games, doing Sudoku and crossword puzzles, learning to play a musical instrument, taking language courses, surfing the internet, and using new brain-enhancing computer games. Partaking in these activities all helps to maintain cognitive ability. In addition, there is solid evidence to show that older people who continue working or who volunteer to help in their communities have better attitudes to ageing and maintain their cognitive skills for longer.

Apart from these conventional approaches to keeping your brain young, there are a few more things you could do to keep your brain flexible, engaged and 'plastic':

- Go to work via a different route to see new sights and stimulate new thoughts.

- Use your non-dominant hand for some tasks that you may have never used it for, like your computer mouse, your hairbrush, stirring a pot on the stove, or eating.

- Eat with chopsticks or with a knife and fork, whichever is not your normal way of eating.

- Have in-depth discussions with people who are experts in their field. You will learn new things and you will ask questions, which is stimulating to your brain.

- Read books that are different from what you're accustomed to.

- Go to a different holiday destination. You will have new travel plans to make, new people to meet and new foods to taste.

Sleep

Sleep is so basic to our lives that most of us never take a moment to think about how weird sleeping actually is. You go to bed every night, lie down and lose awareness of what is going on around you for many hours. When you wake up, if you're lucky enough to sleep all night, you get up and start your life again, only to return to your bed when it's time to lie down again and become unconscious.

It seems that the human brain has a built-in mechanism that promotes alert wakefulness during the day and sleepiness at night. Researchers believe this is why shift workers, who often work through the night, have difficulty establishing and maintaining consistent sleep patterns. In addition, they also suffer significantly more health challenges, including weight gain and obesity. But it's not just about how we are primed to be awake when the sun is shining and sleeping when the sun sets, because sleep is more complex than this.

How much sleep does your brain need?

Most people are sleeping a lot less than they did 50 years ago. Edison's invention of the light bulb in the 1880s changed our approach to the daylight, wake-up/night-time, sleep-time pattern that humans had become accustomed to from the beginning of time.

We now live in a 24/7 world where people are scared they will miss out on something interesting, financially rewarding or fun if they go to bed early. Add shift workers, international travellers, students and work-a-holics to this mix and you have a planet that is continuously pushing the boundaries of physical and mental wellbeing. We have changed a basic, evolutionary urge to suit a modern-day technological phenomenon and this has resulted in changes to our basic health.

Your body evolved to spend one-third of its life asleep — less than that and you end up with health problems. There are a few — very few — unusual people who seem to need less sleep, and researchers believe this is an aberration and definitely not the norm. Each cycle of sleep has a specific function and influences your thinking, immune system, memory, growth and rate of ageing. When you try to squeeze something as important as sleep into a time that suits you and not when your body and brain requires it, you will pay the price of sluggish thinking, poor mood and weight gain. You will not feel light and bright!

Famous dreams

- **Paul McCartney heard the tune for the song 'Yesterday' in a dream.**
- **The book *The Strange Case of Dr Jekyll and Mr Hyde* is based on a dream Robert Louis Stevenson had.**
- **Albert Einstein dreamt about the Theory of Relativity.**
- **The 'Kubla Khan' and 'The Rhyme of the Ancient Mariner' are based on Samuel Taylor Coleridge's dreams.**
- **The entire periodic table is based on a dream by chemist Dmitri Mendeleyev.**
- **The sewing machine needle is the result of a dream Elias Howe had about savages who had holes in the top of their spears.**
- **Golfer Jack Nicklaus changed his swing after a revealing dream.**

Different sleep stages for different brain activities

Sleep is made up of different stages and each performs an important function. Researchers believe each sleep stage accomplishes various tasks in our brain and have to occur to keep the brain healthy. When these stages of sleep are disrupted or you don't get enough sleep, your brain will not be as alert or as capable of learning or remembering things. Your processing speed and accuracy, as well as spatial learning, reaction time and working memory are all influenced negatively. You could also become emotionally unstable. Here are the three basic stages of sleep you should experience every night, which adds up to between seven and eight hours of sleep per night:

1. Shallow sleep occurs as you fall asleep and is also called stage 1 and 2 sleep. During this sleep stage you can be awakened very easily.

2. Deep sleep, or stages 2 and 3 sleep, occurs next. When you move into deep sleep, the parts of your brain that focus on arousal slow down as do the areas involved in controlling muscle movement. The sending of information to consolidate or retrieve memories also slows down considerably, and the alert for sensory information virtually shuts down. Your brain becomes quiet and uses very little energy compared to when you are awake, although laying down the memories of things you learnt during the day continues. This is why researchers believe this type of sleep enhances creativity. During this stage of sleep your energy reserves are replenished. If you are severely sleep deprived, you may not sleep longer when you do go to sleep, but you will experience a lot more of this kind of deep sleep.

3. Rapid eye movement or REM sleep occurs next. This is when you dream, seeing pictures in your mind's eye, because the area of your brain that integrates visual information becomes active. The areas that regulate muscle movement, breathing, heart rate and emotions all become more active as well. Vision, hearing, sensory and memory activity also increase.

Once the first cycle of sleep is complete, it is then repeated, taking between 90 and 120 minutes to go through one whole cycle.

z z z z z

Why our dreams are often odd

During the dream state or REM sleep, the frontal lobes, which help you to think in a logical, sequential manner, slow down their activity markedly. The result is that you are not inhibited by logic or reality when you dream — you can fly, be an angel, revisit your childhood home or live in a different country. Dreams are often ridiculous because our frontal lobes aren't working to make sense of our thoughts. Interestingly, not all animals sleep as we do. Dolphins can shut down half of their brain and continue swimming while sleeping.

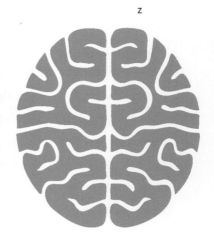

Why do we sleep?

Many researchers have spent considerable time trying to find out why our desire for sleep is so strong and why we get ill and eventually die when we are severely sleep deprived. Looking at what the sleeping brain does has given them clues to follow in this investigation. Allowing the brain to rest and therefore replenish energy stores, lowering the brain's temperature, or enabling the brain to detox are all explanations given as to why sleep is imperative. However, what researchers also discovered is that if you miss a night's sleep, the next night you will have much more REM sleep, which indicates that dreaming is also essential.

Researchers who deprived people of REM sleep discovered that they would be more severely distressed and unable to function properly compared to those deprived of light or deep sleep stages. So, one of the important reasons we sleep is to dream. Why? The areas of the brain that are used during dreaming are not used very often when we are awake. It may be that to keep these areas in working condition, we have to use them in our dreaming. In addition, we may dream to solve problems that are not easily solved using our logical, methodical frontal lobes, but which need a creative, illogical pattern of thinking to be explained.

Other theories about why we sleep include that it reinforces changes in the brain that are produced by our experiences or learning. Sleep helps you to make memories of what you have learnt or experienced during the day. Researchers have found that when you are exposed to a lot of new information or experiences during the day, you will experience more REM sleep. And when you experience more REM sleep, you will also consolidate emotional information from the day more efficiently. Lots of deep sleep will help you to remember and be able to recall a new motor task that you have learnt, while a combination of lots of REM and deep sleep will help you to better retain perceptual information.

Interestingly, when researchers looked at specific neurons involved in learning a new task during the day, they found the same ones were busy during the night in the stage of deep sleep. Sleep may be the time when the brain practises new memory patterns to transfer them into long-term memory. Researchers believe this to be true because there are specific molecular signalling pathways that are sensitive to sleep deprivation. Therefore, sleep could be promoting brain plasticity or facilitating its ability to lay down memories. There are researchers who believe this is not true and they continue to debate this. However, whether sleep helps you to store memories or not, it has some imperative and essential function to perform that is important for your cognitive health.

Another simple explanation given for the benefit of sleeping is that when you sleep, your blood pressure drops. Lowering your blood pressure is good for your heart, and we know that what is good for your heart is also good for your brain. When you work overtime or suffer from insomnia, your heart has to work harder because your blood pressure doesn't drop. As a result, you increase your likelihood of heart disease, which will put your brain at risk for cognitive decline due to a lack of blood flow and, ultimately, oxygen to the brain.

But why else do we sleep? Is it to detoxify the brain? Although our body cells have space around them to flush out toxins and get rid of the accumulated debris that results from cellular activity, our brain does not have the same luxury. How then do our specialized, sophisticated brain cells get rid of accumulated toxins and the by-products of energy production? Through a beautifully organized and very efficient system which relies on sleep.

Just as we have a lymphatic system in the body, the brain has a system called the glymphatic system, which controls the flow of cerebrospinal fluid (CSF), a specialized liquid that surrounds the spinal cord and the brain.

In one study led by Dr Xie, a specific type of dye was injected into the central nervous system (CNS) of a group of mice to see what occurred in the brain when the dye combined with their CSF. At the same time, the researchers monitored their electrical brain activity. When the mice were asleep the dye flowed quickly, but when they were awake, it hardly moved at all. This suggested that the space between brain cells changed depending on whether the mice were asleep or awake. The researchers discovered that the space between their brains cells increased by up to 60 per cent when they were asleep. This allowed the brain fluid to flow around and between neurons with ease. Amazingly, they also found that the accumulated toxic molecules associated with Alzheimer's disease (called beta-amyloid) were flushed away more efficiently when the mice were sleeping.

Even though this research only examined rodent brains, we do know the human brain suffers from sleep deprivation in similar ways to theirs. So, if our brain responds in a similar way, the aim of our glymphatic system is also to initiate CSF flow through the brain when sleep descends to flush toxins and debris out of our brain. In doing so, it clears out the accumulated waste surrounding our neurons.

This research removes many of the questions about sleep and highlights its critically important role in keeping your brain optimally healthy.

How darkness 'speaks' to your brain

Melatonin is a very important neurotransmitter that is produced by the pineal gland, a tiny bean-sized organ that sits in the centre of the brain. The pineal gland responds to light via the eyes. When we see darkness, the message says 'make melatonin' so that we can go to sleep. When we perceive light, a signal is sent to the pineal gland to tell it to stop producing melatonin so that we wake up.

An imbalance in this important hormone means that your day/night or awake/sleep cycle gets disturbed, resulting in unpleasant changes in the ability to fall asleep and feel awake.

Many people simply need to get outside in the daylight to stimulate the pineal gland to start functioning correctly. Spending too much time indoors in unnatural, artificial light can affect the function of the pineal gland. In addition, avoiding artificial light in the evening before sleep allows melatonin levels to rise naturally, which helps your brain to naturally usher in sleep when you get into bed.

Unfortunately, as you get older your production of melatonin declines, which makes it even more important to get outside at the beginning of the day to keep that pineal gland stimulated.

Avoid the news at night!

Avoid stressful experiences as much as possible before bedtime. This means not watching the news in the late evening, or looking over those papers from work, or reading emails and responding to them, as this puts your brain in work mode and not sleep mode. You are fooling yourself if you think you are getting more done by skipping sleep. You may be up and awake, but it's much harder for your brain to focus on what you are doing and to remember what you need it to when it is tired.

Your brain and body need a proper sleep routine, so go to sleep and get up at the same time every day to establish a solid sleep pattern. Ensure that your bedroom is uncluttered and peaceful. It should be a haven, not a stress-den. Eat your main meal early and only have a small snack before bedtime. Keep a notebook on your bedside table to jot down the thoughts that run around your head. It is easier to keep your mind calm and relaxed when you know your plans for the next day are down on paper.

Your brain is an ancient organ and doesn't respond well to the overstimulating and overwhelming world that we have created for ourselves. Respect its desire for peace and calm before sleep, knowing that it will reward you with a rejuvenating sleep. Energized thinking only occurs in a well-rested brain, so you can get ahead in whatever you're trying to accomplish simply by having consistent, good, solid sleep.

Sex and your brain

Sex is a great, natural de-stressor! Being in a fulfilling, happy and satisfying relationship is very good for your brain because humans find companionship both enjoyable and relaxing, which releases neurochemicals and hormones that keep the brain young.

A loving, intimate relationship involves sex, which allows the release of numerous hormones and neurochemicals, such as dopamine, which leaves both partners feeling connected, satisfied and relaxed.

Furthermore, the increased blood flow to the body and sexual organs keeps these tissues and organs healthy, while the brain also receives a boost of extra oxygen and nutrients with the increased blood flow. Sex also strengthens your relationship, which has a de-stressing effect on your brain simply because humans are happier when they are in a relationship with another caring adult. Conversely, being in an unhappy relationship creates stress and will not lead to the kind of sex that makes you happy and relaxed (if you even have sex in this type of relationship!). Dr John Medina, a developmental molecular biologist who has written extensively about how the brain works, has stated that getting into bed at night with your partner, if you are unhappy in your relationship, is like getting into bed with a saber-toothed tiger because adrenaline is released, which arouses you in a very negative way.

Orgasms are better for you than Sudoku!

Recent research has shown that having an orgasm is better for your brain than playing Sudoku. Scientists looked at what happens in the brain when people have sex and then reach an orgasm. During sex the whole brain is involved with various centres including the amygdala and pituitary gland lighting up, regulating emotions and releasing hormones which increase feelings of trust, love and bonding. The increased blood flow and activity recorded in these areas means that there is also increased nutrient supply. The scientists agree that although mental activity is good for the brain and Sudoku is helpful in keeping parts of the brain busy, it only benefits specific areas, whereas orgasms activate the whole brain. Although this research focused on female orgasms, there is nothing to say that there is not a very positive brain effect for men's brains during orgasms too.

In addition, being in an unhappy relationship will cause you to age faster. The hormone cortisol is released when you are unhappy and highly stressed, which stops brain cells (and every other cell in your body) from using and producing energy efficiently. Consequently you age faster on the outside and the inside — artery thickening, inflammation and a lowering of your immune system are the side effects of too much cortisol. Experiencing this challenge on an ongoing basis is very damaging to a brain that desires connection and safety versus anxiety and stress.

Social activity

When you are socially active and engage in many activities that involve relating to others, you are using your brain and keeping it active. This activity is now believed to be very important in keeping your brain stimulated and can also help your neurons to generate new connections.

Interestingly, if you experience loneliness, you have an increased risk of developing dementia. Ongoing friendships and frequent social interactions are integral to cognitive wellbeing. Dr Robert Wilson, the lead author of a four-year longitudinal study, found that negative social interactions are a risk factor for cognitive decline as we age. Often, as people get older, they want their lives to slow down. Many researchers in the field believe this is the worst thing an ageing person can allow to happen. Normal ageing added to inactivity and a negative outlook on life will magnify cognitive decline. In addition, your personality can also affect how your brain ages. The qualities of extraversion and openness contribute to better social, cognitive and physical functioning.

Hormone changes in ageing

Testosterone, estrogen (oestrogen) and progesterone — the so-called sex hormones — gain access to the brain and can therefore trigger various behaviours and feelings. Imbalances of these substances influence behaviour in myriad ways.

Perimenopause is the name given to the phase that precedes menopause in women, which can be as long as ten years. During this time, a woman's ovaries gradually produce less oestrogen. Many women experience various psychological problems, such as mood disturbances and memory challenges, until the cessation of their periods, which is seen as the menopause. Sleep challenges are common during this time. There seems to be a complex relationship between hormones, memory and mood. Many women throughout the world have sought relief from these symptoms by supplementing with HRT (hormone replacement therapy), which is a synthetic form of estrogen. However, the use of bio-identical hormones (via bio-identical hormone replacement therapy or BHRT) is gaining momentum, as the body knows how to use these hormones more effectively.

Men's levels of testosterone begin falling in the early to mid fifties and symptoms include irritability, depression, sleep disruption, anxiety and erectile dysfunction. Unfortunately, the challenges don't stop there as lowered testosterone also influences cognition, although the precise mechanism is not yet understood fully.

The challenge when supplementing hormones to ageing men and women is finding the right balance. Hormones are so specific in their function, and work together so intricately, that it is possible to undermine the delicate balance that the body strives to maintain. When taking hormone supplements, the other ones may become unbalanced because it takes only a very small amount of one hormone to change the way the others work, and change the result of what the supplemented hormone was intended for. A cycle of imbalance could easily be started. In France, bio-identical hormone replacement therapy has been used for many years. Researchers in this field believe that supplementing with this natural form of progesterone can be a very valuable tool for women. One amazing claim for the use of this form of progesterone is that it might lower the risk of dementia, possibly due to progesterone's calming action on cells, which is the opposite of estrogen's stimulating effect. If this is the path that you choose, a qualified doctor can prescribe a high-quality progesterone cream which acts transdermally. Do not confuse this type of cream with wild yam cream, which does not contain any hormone.

Men have also been treated successfully with bio-identical hormone replacement therapy. However, supplementing with these hormones should never be attempted without the guidance of an experienced, qualified physician.

Stress and your brain

Stress is ever-present in the world we live in, however, our brains are only equipped to handle stress for periods of 30–60 seconds; after all, we evolved to either run away very quickly from a threat or we became its next meal. That experience usually didn't last long and the brain returned to normal if we survived.

This stress response is an ancient and very elegant, beautiful and well-orchestrated response for any real, physical danger. It was created through millions of years of evolution to enable us to move away from things that frighten us, or may harm or hurt us. The word 'emotion' is based on the Latin word *motere*, which means 'to move'. The body sees stress as an emergency situation and then makes dramatic adjustments to deal with this perceived emergency. You either have to flee or run away, or fight to get rid of the threat.

Three physical responses to experiencing stress

There are three immediate physical responses to stress related to attention and memory. Firstly, your attention becomes very focused on the thing, person, situation or thought that has caused you to feel stressed and your breathing becomes very rapid and shallow.

Secondly, your brain starts processing information related to this experience very quickly, but this speed is counteracted by a severe loss of accuracy in the processing.

Thirdly, your capacity to store any memory in your short-term storage area is reduced. This explains why when you are stressed you are unable to remember where you put your car keys, who you were just introduced to, or what you should be doing in front of the cupboards that you find yourself standing in front of. Your attention is only focused on your stressor, your brain is working like crazy but not very well, and your hippocampus, where your memories are created and stored, is having a little break.

Interestingly, although you wouldn't notice this effect on yourself, your eyes also start moving more rapidly when you are anxious, supposedly to increase your ability to search for solutions to stress-induced situations.

Of course, there are many neurochemicals that start working their way through your body and brain too.

Ongoing stress and your memory

Ongoing, unrelenting stress exerts an insidious but devastating effect on brain function, ultimately leading to cognitive decline, particularly in relation to memory.

Memory is made up of three main components: seeing, doing and listening. When these are all present, memory has an easy task embedding its chemicals in the right places for good recall. When you are stressed this whole process doesn't work properly, so you end up forgetting things. The specific part of memory that is regularly seen by researchers to decline in the ageing brain is the type that deals with personal facts, such as what you ate for breakfast and where you went last weekend. This type of memory is called episodic memory and can be formed from both short- and long-term memories.

Ongoing stress and your adrenal glands

Adrenaline is produced very quickly in the adrenal glands when a threat is perceived. It is powerful and short-lived, resulting in increased heart rate and dilated pupils while blood is pushed into the muscles, heart and brain to deal with the threat. This effect can last up to an hour, after which cortisol kicks in.

Cortisol is another stress-related hormone, and although it's also produced in the adrenal glands, it is slower to get going but its effects last much longer — it's there for when you need a sustained effort to get away from the threat. It helps to get glucose into the muscles, heart and brain to sustain the effort of defeating the threat. However, cortisol stays in the system much longer than adrenaline and gives the brain, especially the hippocampus, a destructive toxic bath.

When you experience stress for an extended period of time, your adrenal glands become exhausted. The nutrients that are required to keep them functioning will become depleted and therefore not be available for many other tasks.

The adrenal glands create hormones, such as adrenaline, cortisol and noradrenaline, which are regulating hormones that respond to the demands that stress places on them. The nutrients that become depleted over time are vitamin C, vitamin E, the B group of vitamins (especially vitamins B3, B5 and B6), magnesium and other trace minerals such as zinc, manganese, selenium, molybdenum, chromium, copper and iodine. These nutrients are essential for so many other functions in the brain that a lack of them will create severe physical and cognitive energy decline, with the resultant increase in anxiety and depression and a decrease in memory ability.

If this wasn't bad enough, researchers have found that the minerals chromium, copper, iron, zinc and especially magnesium are excreted via urine when stress hormones are produced. So, the more stressed you are, the less of these important nutrients you have available to help manage the stress.

Ongoing stress and your digestive system

When you experience ongoing stress, your digestive system becomes compromised, ultimately leading to a reduction in nutrient absorption. Even if you are eating an optimal diet (which is very unusual for most people), due to cravings, blood glucose fluctuations and other stress-induced poor eating habits, the absorption of nutrients is still severely compromised. Supplementation with specific nutrients, such as those mentioned above, can improve both your quality of life and digestive challenges, while you are working to reduce your stress levels (see page 49 for more about stress and digestion, and pages 50–1 for more information about using supplements to aid digestion).

The long-term effects of ongoing stress

A natural side effect of the brain producing excessive quantities of stress hormones is a decrease in the feel-good ones, such as serotonin, dopamine and melatonin. Although there is a natural feedback loop that should switch off the stress response after a threat, ongoing stress makes this loop less and less efficient so that eventually it doesn't switch off properly.

The long-term effects of stress are insidious and not always noticed or felt immediately. The following are the known effects of long-term, ongoing stress:

- immunity suppression

- insulin resistance with high blood sugar and high insulin levels

- high blood pressure

- decrease in serotonin

- increase in norepinephrine

- decrease in thyroid hormones

- neuronal damage and cognitive decline

- slow metabolism

- increased anxiety

- emotional eating

- insomnia

- increased compulsive behaviour

- depression, irritability, anger, emotional instability, anxiety, fear and restlessness

- low energy

- low sexual energy

- decreased fertility

- digestive difficulties

- increased inflammation

- reduced ability to focus and concentrate on a task

- low sex hormone production.

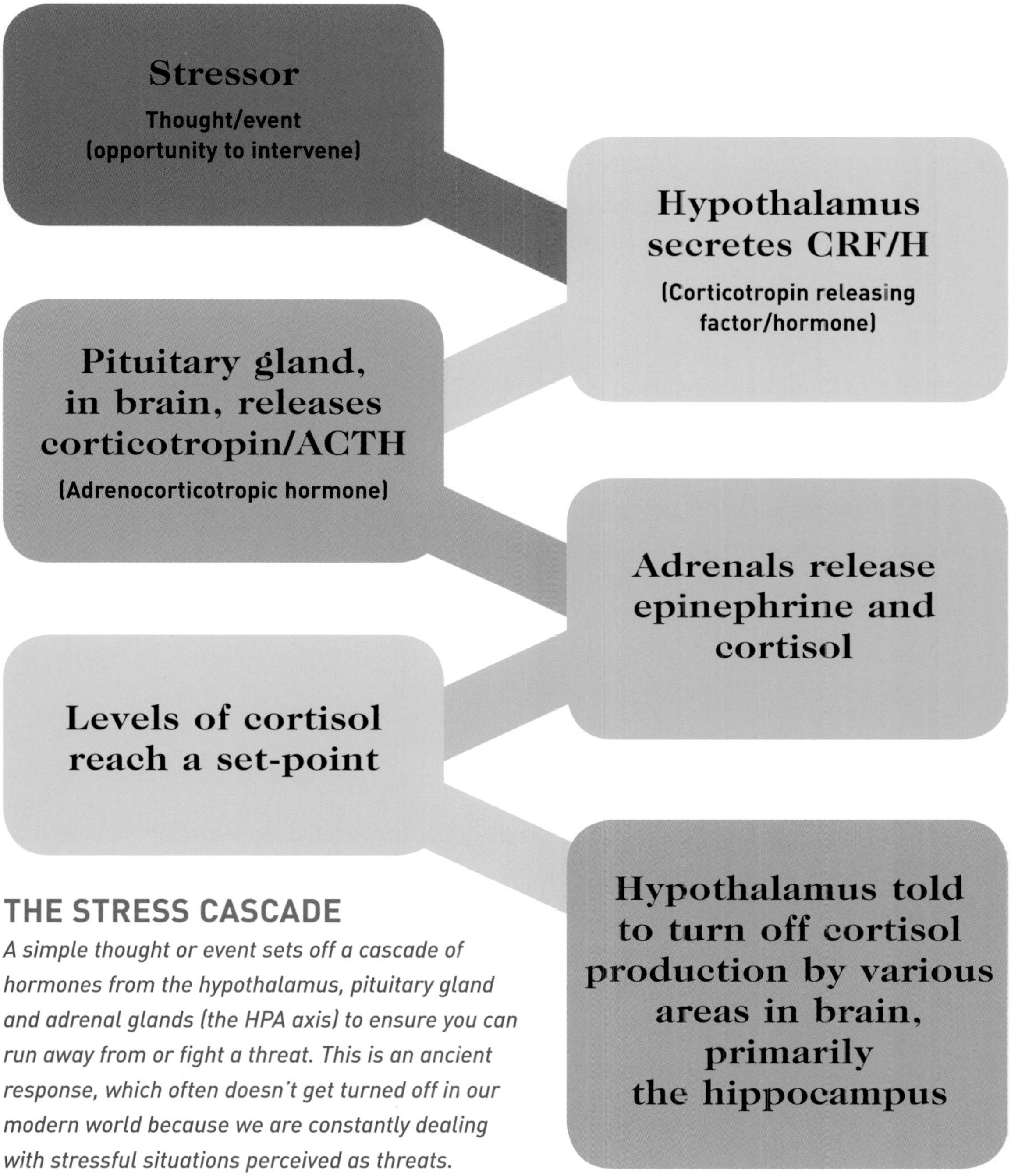

Stressor

**Thought/event
(opportunity to intervene)**

**Hypothalamus
secretes CRF/H**

**(Corticotropin releasing
factor/hormone)**

**Pituitary gland,
in brain, releases
corticotropin/ACTH**

(Adrenocorticotropic hormone)

**Adrenals release
epinephrine and
cortisol**

**Levels of cortisol
reach a set-point**

THE STRESS CASCADE

*A simple thought or event sets off a cascade of
hormones from the hypothalamus, pituitary gland
and adrenal glands (the HPA axis) to ensure you can
run away from or fight a threat. This is an ancient
response, which often doesn't get turned off in our
modern world because we are constantly dealing
with stressful situations perceived as threats.*

**Hypothalamus told
to turn off cortisol
production by various
areas in brain,
primarily
the hippocampus**

Multi-tasking is a myth

Multi-tasking is not possible, as your brain is only capable of truly focusing on one thing at a time. It uses its unique ability to focus, with awareness, to complete one task well. When you try to accomplish too many things at the same time your brain feels stressed, which increases your levels of cortisol and actually further diminishes your brain's ability to cope with stress and accomplish tasks effectively. And women are no better at multi-tasking than men — that's another myth based on the fact that women's brains are generally more active at any one time than men's.

Why does stress feel so much worse right now?

There are very few people in the world right now who feel calm, cool and collected. It seems as if we have created huge problems for ourselves and they seem insurmountable.

There are three elements related to the stress that we are experiencing, that seem to produce the greatest threat to our wellbeing:

1. lack of predictability

2. lack of control, and

3. lack of obvious outlets for the resultant frustration.

The stress that you experience in relation to these three elements is usually perceived as being larger than it actually is. Stress involving these three components is 'uncontrolled stress' and generally continues for a prolonged period of time due to your inability to control it. Even if it isn't severe, it is more dangerous to your cognitive health than a short-term incident of a major stress because of this perceived lack of control.

This is, of course, the worst kind of stress for the brain to experience, as it works best and is more creative when it is calm and relaxed, yet alert. So in order to solve our challenges, we should try to keep our brain relaxed. To maintain this balance is very difficult in the modern world, but it is something that is worth striving for.

A calm mind leads to a healthier brain

Research has shown that practising meditation and focusing on compassion over a number of years strengthens the emotional regions of the brain. The brains of Buddhist monks were compared to people performing meditation for the first time, with the results showing that the years of consistent meditation practice had changed the structure of the monks' brains while the inexperienced subjects displayed no difference in the same brain regions. The connections between the thinking and feeling regions of the monks' brains were strong. Their ability to regulate their emotions was also highly developed. In addition, other research showed that long-term practitioners of meditation have a larger right hippocampus, a brain region responsible for response control as well as emotional regulation. People practising meditation do exhibit emotional stability, engage in mindful behaviour and cultivate positive emotions — all characteristics that this region of the hippocampus is involved in. There is also a link between long-term practitioners and positive cardio-respiratory control, which can explain some of the positive effects that they experience. In another study, the meditation practitioners were found to have a lower age-related decline in the thickness of specific cortical regions in the brain, which is wonderful news. Your cortex is where your higher reasoning and planning takes place. However, the benefits of meditation are not just linked to the production of new neurons, better reasoning and emotional control, or better breathing, but also to the quality of life one experiences when feeling calmer, more in control and able to withstand the negative effects of stress.

Action plan

Five things to do that will introduce more sweat, sleep and sex into your life and decrease stress:

1. Find someone to exercise with to help hold you accountable, and set a date to exercise at least three times a week.

2. Find a new activity that will absorb your time and attention for at least five hours a week — volunteering is a good idea as it allows you to focus on something outside yourself.

3. If you suffer from poor sleep, look at ways to improve your sleep patterns and persevere until you find the solution.

4. Get committed to improving a bad relationship, or leave a bad relationship.

5. Evaluate your life seriously and simplify it enough for you to feel calm most of the time. A very effective way to start doing this is to make time for meditation and calm reflection to slow down your busy brain.

See the Resources section for more supportive information.

CHAPTER 2

What food intolerances do to your brain

A healthy brain starts with good nutrition. Food enters your body via your mouth and requires proper chewing for the digestive process to begin. Once inside your stomach, the food must be broken down into tiny particles with help from digestive enzymes and stomach acid. As these food particles travel through the digestive tract, they need to be absorbed through the cells lining the intestine and transported through blood vessels into the bloodstream so the body gets all the nutrients it needs for optimal functioning. It is imperative that your digestive system is functioning well so you absorb all the nutrients your body needs from food. Once in the bloodstream, these essential nutrients cross the blood–brain barrier into brain tissue, helping your brain to function at its best.

For your brain to function optimally, it needs fuel in the form of glucose, essential fats, protein, vitamins and minerals. Your brain needs the right proteins and fats, as well as specific nutrients to enable it to grow new connections. This is done by eating the right foods and avoiding the ones that could be causing you digestive distress. Without these building blocks, the brain won't work properly, and the effects are felt as negative ripples throughout your life.

Unfortunately, many people disregard food while they pursue a busy lifestyle. They tend to eat too many chemically laden, highly processed foods that are deficient in the very nutrients the brain needs to work optimally and contain compounds that actually damage the brain. As a result, obesity levels are at an all-time high, which is now also linked to the high rates of depression and stress found across most cultures and socio-economic levels. Food allergies and intolerances are rising too, leaving us to conclude that certain foods do not suit our body or our brain.

The aim of this chapter is to give you a clear understanding of the foods that are related to food allergies and intolerances. I will explain what they do to the brain (and body) and give you a clear idea of how to improve your digestion.

The difference between food allergy and food intolerance

An allergy is a physical response to a substance where the immune system is clearly involved. The responses are immediate and often life-threatening. They involve respiratory difficulties, skin rashes, a drop in blood pressure, an irregular heartbeat, and in severe cases, loss of consciousness. The test for this type of allergy is the IgE test, which measures the levels of immunoglobulin E antibodies produced when the immune cells are exposed to a particular substance. The E can be a reminder that this type of allergy represents an 'Emergency'.

A food intolerance or sensitivity to a particular food is where there is no measurable antibody response. For example, someone who is unable to digest the sugar in milk (lactose) can develop mild abdominal discomfort when they drink milk, or an intolerance to MSG can produce hyperactivity. The response may not be immediate as it is not an immunoglobulin E allergy response.

The most common type of food intolerance or sensitivity is where there is a delayed reaction to a food because it can take anywhere from an hour to three days for a reaction to manifest. The IgG test (called an enzyme-linked immunosorbent assay) focuses on the amount of immunoglobulin G antibodies produced when your body is exposed to a particular food or foods. The cells that produce IgG antibodies have a half-life of about six weeks, which means that after six weeks half of them remain. The cells have a 'memory' of these antibodies, which is short-term. After about three months they will have 'forgotten' about the food, so re-introducing it should not produce a negative result. However, it is wise to not consume the particular food more than once every four days in an attempt to stop a sensitivity or intolerance from occurring again.

The IgA test measures how many immunoglobulin A antibodies are present in your immune system. These specific antibodies are very important in protecting the mucosal lining of the digestive tract as well as the mouth, nose and genital–urinary tract. Elevated IgA antibodies may be a sign that there is mucous membrane damage present in the gut, which could be caused by ongoing exposure to foods that you are intolerant to, as well as stress, alcohol and certain medications.

If you suspect you may be intolerant to many foods and chemicals, get assessed by a qualified naturopath or nutrition-minded physician, who may suggest a blood test to find out which foods are causing the distress. You may also want to invest in a diary and write down the foods that you eat every day and list any reactions to foods as they appear. Once you decipher which foods are possibly causing you problems, you can begin to narrow down the offenders. Start by avoiding the suspect foods for six weeks and then re-introduce them through a system of rotation, so that you only eat one of them every four days. That way you can determine which food is causing a reaction.

It is important to recognize that you may be regularly eating a food that you are intolerant to without even knowing it because these foods are usually widely consumed. Because there is no immediate response, you may be unaware of the fact that a particular food does not agree with you. Using a food diary can be very helpful to track reactions that you may have been unaware of.

Following is a list of the most common foods that people can be allergic to, but which can also be foods that people are intolerant to:

- wheat (and other gluten grains such as rye and barley. Although oats do not contain gluten, they do contain avenin, a similar substance that can also trigger an immune response in susceptible people.)

- dairy products (milk, cheese etc., especially from cows)
- chocolate
- corn
- eggs
- fish (including shellfish)
- berries
- legumes (soya beans, green peas, lima beans and peanuts)
- nuts
- pork
- peaches.

Other common foods that can cause reactions are oranges, yeast-containing foods and members of the nightshade family — tomatoes, capsicums (bell peppers), potatoes and eggplant (aubergine).

The brain is the most delicate organ in the human body, so it may respond negatively to specific foods (or chemicals or additives in foods) because food influences hormones, neurochemicals and other key nutrients in the body. Any compound that irritates the brain or stops it from operating efficiently will eventually lead to neurological challenges. It may take time, sometimes decades, but the damage will be taking place, slowly but surely.

The chemicals found in additives coupled with foods that you may be intolerant to, have been implicated in various neurological symptoms:

- depression
- headaches
- fatigue, apathy and lethargy
- sleeplessness
- feelings of indecision
- moodiness
- emotional instability

- impaired concentration and mental lapses
- paranoid thinking
- nervousness.

These symptoms are real. Many people have simply learnt to live with them as they do not know what feeling good and symptom-free is like. Why? Because many of the foods available to us today, especially in processed form, are the very foods provoking these symptoms. And because most people have been eating these foods since birth, these symptoms have become 'normal' for them. So feeling light and bright is a foreign concept because their brain has always felt sluggish and slow, unable to sustain a good mood or effective cognitive focus.

What is causing the reaction?

Most food allergies and intolerances are a reaction to the protein in the food. This can be due to an inherited allergy or to a digestive challenge whereby the offending protein isn't being broken down properly by the digestive system. A lack of stomach acid (hydrochloric acid) could also be the problem, which has further repercussions, as many nutrients aren't absorbed adequately when stomach acid is low. Deficiencies in zinc, calcium, as well as vitamin B12, are all due to low stomach acid production. Furthermore, low stomach acid leads to increased food allergies as the body will not recognize the strange, undigested food particle and will therefore mount an attack.

In addition, if you have taken a lot of antibiotics recently, your digestive tract may have become crowded with bad bacteria and lost too many good bacteria, leading to a predisposition to allergies. This is because the lining of your digestive tract has become 'leaky' and allows large particles of food to cross into the bloodstream, causing the body to respond negatively because it doesn't recognize these large food molecules.

How do you know if you are intolerant to a food?

One of the quickest ways to find out if a food is jeopardizing your chances of feeling cognitively alert and leading to unstable moods is to check the following four points:

1. Are you obsessed with a certain food? Arranging your life in such a way to ensure you obtain this food is a sure sign of an addiction to the specific food.

2. Will you eat the food that you are obsessed with even if you suffer from negative consequences when you eat it? Many people still eat specific foods knowing that they will feel bloated, irritable and generally miserable after eating them.

3. Do you experience lack of control when you start eating the food? Is one serving never enough? An inability to stop the behaviour or to control it is a sign that you could very well be addicted to the food in question.

4. Do you deny that the food you eat so regularly could be causing a problem? If you refuse to admit that the food in question could be responsible for your moodiness, bloated stomach, headaches or weepiness, then you could very well be intolerant to it.

Another clear sign of food intolerance is dark circles under the eyes. Why? Food intolerances can cause nasal congestion, which causes the veins that drain from your eyes to your nose to darken and dilate. Pollens and airborne irritants can have the same effect.

In addition, the physical reactions to food intolerances such as bloating, headaches, frequent infections, sinusitis, skin rashes, joint pain, constipation and/or diarrhoea, as well as a lack of energy are clear signs that your food choices are not supporting optimal health. A leaky gut is unfortunately one of the outcomes of the long-term consumption of foods that you are intolerant to (see page 49 for more on the leaky gut).

The science of addiction

Endorphins are chemical messengers the brain produces to reduce pain. They also produce feelings of wellbeing and pleasure. Morphine, heroin and cocaine all stimulate the production of vast quantities of endorphins, which leads to feelings of euphoria. Feeling very scared, such as when you watch a horror movie (now you know why some people are addicted to them), and having an orgasm also produce endorphins in the brain. Exercise is another way to produce endorphins, while eating certain foods such as hot chillies can do the same thing.

Sugar also causes the release of endorphins in the brain, leading to an association between sugar and pleasant feelings. In this way, eating sugar-laden foods becomes an endorphin-rush activity, one that has to be repeated regularly to keep the endorphins circulating. If you have learnt that you get an endorphin rush from these types of food, it is very likely that you will repeat this behaviour.

Manufacturers of processed and refined carbohydrates have spent billions of dollars on discovering exactly what people like to eat. Scientists came up with the term 'mouth feel' to describe the complex interactions of food texture and taste, as well as the way the food feels in the mouth and what taste lingers in the mouth and on the tongue after the food is swallowed. Various additives such as gums, stabilizers, emulsifiers and starches can be added to food to produce the mouth feel consumers want.

A specific machine called the TA.XT*Plus* Texture Analyzer, which is essentially an artificial mouth, analyses data from 25 different probes to assess the properties of the foods such as bounce, crunchiness, lumpiness, smoothness, softness and 'spread-ability'. In addition, the release of endorphins, as discussed earlier, makes the addiction to specific mouth-feel foods even more complex.

Food addiction

Exorphins have a similar action to endorphins but they come into the body from an external source, hence their name. They are small fragments of protein (peptides) that result from the breakdown of specific foods. Gluten as well as dairy products produce exorphins.

Gluten is the common name for a protein found in wheat, rye and barley. It is also found in other more ancient forms of grass-like cereals such as spelt, kamut and triticale. Gluten performs an important function in these grass grains by helping to protect and germinate the seed to ensure its survival. It is therefore a very tough and resilient protein and difficult to digest. Gluten, when broken down in the digestive tract, contains compounds with a mild opiate effect (gluteomorphin – a type of exorphin). It would seem that an interaction between the immune system and gluten may lead to blood vessel damage in the brain, which leads to the psychological and behavioural disturbances that gluten-sensitive people experience such as depression, mood disorders and severe irritability. Increased intestinal permeability is also thought to play a significant role in these symptoms, as there is a direct path from the gut into the bloodstream for gluteomorphins. Celiac patients, who suffer an autoimmune response to gluten, have been known to suffer from a wide range of neurological disturbances, some of which have involved changes to the structure of the brain.

Dairy foods include milk, yoghurt and cheese as well as many processed foods such as dried milk powder, milk protein and whey. It is possible to be allergic or intolerant to either the lactose (milk sugar) or the casein (milk protein) in dairy. Most mammals, including humans, stop producing the enzyme lactase, which breaks down lactose, after weaning. Cheese, a concentrated source of protein and fat, contains trace amounts of casomorphin (an exorphin), which has a similar action to morphine. Whether these casomorphins make their way into our bloodstream is still under debate, although researchers suggest that some of them do, reaching their peak 40 minutes after ingestion. It may simply be that the combination of protein and fats is addictive because these are such important foods from a survival perspective. Cheese also contains PEA (phenylethylamine), which harbours traces of a compound similar to THC (tetrahydrocannabinol), which is the active ingredient in marijuana. Chocolate also contains PEA. In addition, cheese is often salty, which is an additive that is easy to get addicted to.

Your brain and gut are directly linked

It should come as no surprise to you that your brain and your gut are intricately connected. The food that you eat has to be digested and absorbed to sustain optimal brain function. If anything disturbs the digestive and absorption process (as well as the elimination process), cognitive function will suffer.

Most people today eat too many processed foods and very little raw food. The digestive enzymes found in raw food help your digestive system break food down into tiny particles that can be absorbed and used by your body. The fewer enzymes you have in your diet from raw foods, the less effective your digestive system will be. When there is a lack of digestive enzymes in your diet, two problems occur:

1. Undigested fragments of food can be absorbed through the digestive tract straight into the bloodstream. As a result, antibodies in the bloodstream recognize these particles as foreign invaders and mount an attack against them. This creates an inflammatory reaction within the body.

2. The digestion of protein is severely limited when there are not enough digestive enzymes, which is of real concern, because protein is the foundation of hormones (such as leptin and insulin), which keep blood levels stable. Unstable blood glucose has been linked to moodiness, depression, anxiety and weight gain. Protein is also the basis of many of the neurotransmitters required to keep the brain working well. Obviously, an imbalance in the neurotransmitters sets the stage for poor mental health and ongoing poor food choices, leading to a downward spiral of unstable moods, poor concentration and lowered memory potential.

The 'leaky' gut

Digestive challenges are often the underlying factor in food intolerances. The digestive tract can become 'leaky' due to a number of reasons, including excessive antibiotic use, a deficiency in important nutrients (for example essential fats, zinc, vitamin A), ongoing inflammation, an imbalance of gut bacteria, and stress.

This 'leakiness' means that partially digested proteins enter the bloodstream and trigger a reaction from the immune system. Part of the solution to food intolerant reactions is to get the digestive system working properly again by firstly removing the foods that are causing the reactions, and then adding the right nutrients into the diet such as essential fats, zinc, probiotics and digestive enzymes. Ensuring that your diet includes plenty of fresh fruit and vegetables, as well as clean forms of protein and unrefined carbohydrates is critically important too.

Unfortunately, stress is another huge reason for digestive challenges. Digestion naturally stops when you are extremely stressed because the body doesn't want to waste time digesting food when it senses that you are fighting for survival. Your brain doesn't know that the stress may not be life-threatening. This results in stagnating food sitting in your digestive tract and a build-up of toxins, as well as stress hormones interfering with digestion. Less severe stress also results in digestive challenges because the same stress hormones interfere with optimal digestion and also damage the gut lining. In addition, when people are stressed, they often eat more in an attempt to alleviate the feelings of distress. This obviously adds to the digestive disaster. It is better to eat small, nutrient-dense meals when you are experiencing stress.

Benefits of digestive enzymes and probiotics

When your food is chewed properly and then digested well, it can be absorbed optimally. When this happens your brain gets the nutrients it requires and your body can work well too. When it doesn't work well your mood, memory, learning and ability to focus all suffer. We know now that a lot of what goes on in the gut influences the brain directly because some neurotransmitters, like serotonin, are actually more plentiful in the gut than they are in the brain. Recent research has linked the digestive system to psychiatric conditions, leading to a new understanding and appreciation of how the gut and the brain are connected.

Using digestive enzymes helps your gut to break down food into its working components and facilitate optimal digestion. For example, a good store-bought digestive enzyme contains protease to help digest protein, lipase to digest fat and amylase to digest carbohydrates. Maltase, which converts complex sugars from grains into glucose, phytase which helps with overall digestion, and cellulase which helps digest cellulose (the fibre found in plant foods) are also good additions. If you experience bloating, heartburn, gas, acid reflux or nausea, these are signs that your digestive system is not working optimally. Stress, inflammation and ageing all influence the body's ability to produce enough digestive enzymes to digest food. Supplementing with a good digestive enzyme and increasing the amount of raw or lightly steamed foods you eat will enhance your digestive processes and positively influence your brain's ability to work optimally. Always take digestive enzymes with a meal and see a medical practitioner if your digestive system has been bothering you for some time.

We also need good gut bacteria to help our digestive tract work at its best. These good bacteria are damaged and reduced in number when our food is highly processed, when we are stressed and when we do not digest our food adequately. Antibiotic use also depletes these good bacteria. The end result is poor digestion and inflammation in the gut.

Adding a good probiotic to your diet helps your digestive system work optimally and reduces inflammation, which will influence brain health positively. A good store-bought probiotic (which you will find in the refrigerated section of health food stores) can start the process of re-colonizing your digestive tract with good or 'gut-friendly' bacteria. The best strains are from the *Lactobacillus* genus and the *acidophilus*, *rhamnosus* and *plantarum* species. Probiotics are produced commercially by allowing the good bacteria to grow in a safe environment and then 'harvesting' them into capsules that we can use. Live cultured yoghurt is a natural way to get digestive enzymes and probiotics into your daily diet. Choose coconut yoghurt if you want to avoid dairy, but be sure to read the labels of any yoghurt you choose to use, as many are loaded with sugars as well as artificial sweeteners and flavours. Fermented foods such as kimchi, sauerkraut and pickles also contain probiotics, but be sure to choose ones made with brine and not vinegar. The popular drink kombucha is also a good source of probiotics.

Adding a prebiotic, which provides food for probiotics, will ensure that the good bacteria in your gut keep working optimally. Prebiotics can be found naturally in asparagus, leeks and onions, Jerusalem artichokes and chicory (Belgian endive), burdock and dandelion roots. Cabbage, cauliflower, Brussels sprouts, kale and radishes are also good sources.

Naturally occurring chemicals that can cause cognitive challenges

Even though a food is 'natural' that does not mean it is chemical-free. All foods are made up of chemicals, although the combination of chemicals found in natural, unprocessed foods are generally less challenging to our health. Some people are sensitive to the natural chemicals found in food, mainly salicylates, amines and benzoates, often experiencing hyperactivity, insomnia, compulsive behaviour and depression as side effects.

Salicylates are natural chemicals found in plants, which protect them from pests and diseases. The best-known salicylate is aspirin, which comes from the bark of the willow tree. If you are sensitive to aspirin, you are likely to be sensitive to salicylates too. Salicylates give food a zesty, sharp, tangy flavour. While a single dose doesn't do much harm to someone who is sensitive to salicylates, when exposed to them many times a day, the effects slowly build up causing various symptoms such as hyperactivity, skin rashes or digestive challenges. The IgG test does not pick up salicylate sensitivity.

Salicylates are commonly used to add flavour to foods, usually in much higher doses than they are found in nature. They are found in a wide variety of foods (see below), so can be difficult to eliminate. The salicylate content of fruits and vegetables increases with ripening.

As the following list contains many nutritious foods, it wouldn't be wise to cut them all out, nor would it be easy. This should only be attempted under the guidance of a qualified naturopath or a nutrition-minded physician. Salicylates also inhibit the conversion and use of essential fats, so it may help to increase the supply of these healthy fats in your diet too.

FOODS CONTAINING SALICYLATES

almonds	licorice
apples	macadamia nuts
berries	mint, peppermint
broccoli	mushrooms
capsicum (bell pepper)	olives
cherries	pineapples
chicory (Belgian endive)	pine nuts (pine kernels)
	pistachio nuts
citrus fruit	radishes
dried fruit	raspberries
gherkins (pickles)	spices
grapes	tea
guavas	tomatoes
herbs	watercress
kiwi fruit	Worcestershire sauce

Amines are a group of chemicals that occur both in the body and brain, as well as naturally in many foods, and may cause allergic reactions that can lead to cognitive difficulties. The level of amines increases as the food ripens. The enzyme that breaks these chemicals down in the body can be inhibited when certain drugs called monoamine oxidase inhibitors (MAOIs) are being taken. The optimal production of these enzymes can also be hampered by a genetic variant, which could lead to aggression, particularly in men. The IgG test does not pick up sensitivity to these substances either.

Amines are broken down into a few categories, which include histamine, tyramine and phenylethylamine (PEA). These three are discussed below because of their link to mental health challenges and physical reactions.

Histamine is an important neurotransmitter but it is also involved in allergic reactions and the immune system, defending us against dangerous bacteria and viruses. Very high and very low levels of histamine have both been associated with mental health challenges. Very high levels are linked to addictions, abnormal fears, hyperactivity, obsessions, insomnia, emotional instability and schizophrenia. Conversely, very low levels are associated with anxiety, paranoia and hallucinations. Histamine levels in the body are influenced by certain foods which either contain naturally occurring histamine or which stimulate its release. The presence of histadine, an amino acid found in some protein foods that is the precursor for histamine, will also influence histamine levels.

FOODS CONTAINING HISTAMINE

beer	sauerkraut, kimchi, pickles, soya bean sauce, miso, balsamic vinegar and kombucha
cheese	
chocolate	
eggplant (aubergine)	
egg white, raw	fish and shellfish – unless freshly caught, gutted and cooked and eaten within half an hour
fermented foods and sauces, such as	

meat sausages, such as bologna, salami, pepperoni	tea
	tomatoes
pumpkin	vinegar
spinach	wine
strawberries	

Tyramine can lead to severe headaches, feelings of light-headedness as well as itchy, hot flushes in people who are sensitive to it.

FOODS CONTAINING TYRAMINE

avocados	meat extracts, such as Oxo, Bovril
bananas	peanuts
broad beans (fava beans)	raspberries
aged cheeses such as blue cheese, Gruyère, Parmesan, Manchego, Roquefort and Pecorino	red plums
	salted, smoked or pickled fish, especially herring
chicken liver	sour cream
eggplant (aubergine)	tomatoes
fermented foods and sauces, such as sauerkraut, kimchi, pickles, soya bean sauce, miso, balsamic vinegar and kombucha	wine, especially red wine
	yeast extracts, such as Marmite, Vegemite
meat sausages, such as bologna, salami, pepperoni	

Phenylethylamine (PEA) is found in high levels in chocolate, several cheeses and red wine. It is produced in the body from its precursor phenylalanine, and is sometimes referred to as the body's natural amphetamine because it is a natural stimulant and mood enhancer. In large quantities (and for some people, in small quantities), it can produce intense headaches, dizziness, insomnia and confusion. Its presence in chocolate has led people to call it the 'the food of love'.

Benzoic acid is a white, crystalline compound used as a food preservative. It can have a narcotic effect on the brain in very high concentrations, obviously adversely affecting brain function. It can also cause skin breakouts, such as eczema. Benzoates occur naturally in some foods at varying levels, and are particularly high in the following foods. Sodium benzoate is a derivative of benzoic acid and is a commercially prepared preservative, found in processed foods.

FOODS CONTAINING BENZOIC ACID

anise	prunes
cinnamon	raspberries
cloves	strawberries
cranberries	tea
nutmeg	

Why it is not simple to pinpoint food intolerance

Unfortunately, it is not always a simple process to ascertain whether you have a problem with a food or a chemical in a food. It's a process of elimination and once you are aware of the fact that food and various chemicals in foods can have a serious effect on your brain, you become more aware of what foods you love, crave and seemingly can't live without. Often this is the very food that needs to be eliminated from your diet. Using a food diary or working with a nutritionist can also help you to identify an offending food.

Over time, you will learn what you should avoid eating and will also become aware of what substitutes are available. If you get an IgG test, it may give you a good idea of which foods to avoid. However, the chemicals in foods are more difficult to pinpoint, so they will have to be deciphered through a process of elimination and observation. Many people are simply unable to tolerate the vast quantity of unnatural chemicals that pervade processed foods, so when you eliminate them from your pantry, you immediately have less of a toxic load and your brain will naturally start functioning more efficiently, leading to more stable moods and improved cognitive ability.

There is no need for you to feel deprived if you do make the decision to remove a food or a variety of foods from your diet. There are many replacements for the most common foods that cause reactions, although you do have to be careful that they are not overly processed. Read the labels of these replacement foods as carefully as you would any other processed food, as unnecessary additives are not required and may cause further challenges in your diet. There are, unfortunately, many replacement foods that are filled with loads of sugar, other refined carbohydrates, damaging fats, flavourings and preservatives, so it's up to you to search for the best options.

Your ability to flourish and maintain stable moods, to enjoy enhanced learning and good recall are all impacted negatively when your brain is battling to cope with a substance that is causing it distress. By removing a suspect food from your diet for a period of three to four weeks, you will be able to note any changes in mood, focus, concentration and memory. It is best to undergo this elimination diet under the guidance of an expert in food allergies, who will be able to help you eliminate all the possibly offending foods and guide you in choosing suitable alternatives. They will also direct you to the best blood tests available, such as the IgG test, to see which foods could be causing the reactions. For more information go to the Resources section.

Action plan

Five things to do that will highlight and prevent potential allergens in your diet and improve digestive health are:

1. Eating the same foods every day eventually exhausts the body's ability to digest them properly, which can increase the chances of developing food allergies or intolerances. Try to make your diet as varied as possible. Avoiding processed foods is a necessary part of eliminating possible food intolerances and improving digestive health.

2. If you suspect you have a food intolerance, remove gluten and dairy from your diet for one month and assess your moods, focus and concentration as well as digestive health. Introduce them back into your diet separately to determine whether one or both of these foods is causing you digestive distress. Whenever you eliminate a suspected problem food, do it separately so you can determine which food could possibly be causing a reaction.

3. Increase the quantity of fresh, raw vegetables you consume. If your digestion is really impaired, steam your vegetables. If you want to keep on eating raw salads, make sure you are chewing the green leaves and vegetables very well.

4. Add a digestive enzyme to your meals simply by sprinkling the opened capsule over your food (it is tasteless) or swallow the capsule with water during your meal. You can also stir the enzymes into a smoothie.

5. Add a probiotic to your daily routine, after a meal, which reduces the possibility of the good bacteria being destroyed by stomach acid. After dinner is the ideal time as the probiotic has all night to get to work. There are different types of probiotics and a qualified naturopath or nutrition-minded physician can guide you in choosing the right one for your digestive challenge.

See the Resources section for more information.

CHAPTER 3

Why food additives are bad for your brain

Processed foods contain an enormous amount of additives including emulsifiers, stabilizers, flavourings, colourings, damaging fats, various forms of sugar and preservatives. There are over 10,000 chemicals used in the food industry today to produce processed food that is tastier, more colourful and of course 'fresh'. Many of these chemicals are added to food to change its colour — making it more appealing to children — and to preserve its shelf life and keep fats emulsified. Other additives enhance the texture of the food. A number of synthetic vitamins are added to fool consumers into believing that they are actually eating nutritious foods. This practice is more of an advertising and marketing ploy.

Without preservatives, processed food would spoil. Without artificial colours, processed food would look unappetizing. Without artificial flavourings, processed food would not be as tasty. Without various other chemicals, this type of food would lose its texture. Obviously, some of these additives are necessary to keep consumers safe from spoiled food. However, the bottom line is that without additives the food industry couldn't survive, but these additives may be doing real harm to your sensitive brain.

Although household cleaning products and body care products are not foods, they influence brain function due to the toxic chemicals they contain. It is important to know that many of these toxic chemicals can be absorbed into the body through the skin.

The aim of this chapter is to give you a clear idea of what additives do to your brain, whether they come from foods or household and body care products. It will outline the products which are especially harmful and which ones are safe.

The fastest guide to reading labels

All ingredients in food products are now listed according to their prominence, so whatever ingredient is first on the list will comprise most of the product. This is where you may be surprised when you see that 'strawberry jam' actually contains very little strawberry, as it's near the bottom of the ingredient list. Any product with more than five ingredients, unless it is for example an organic tomato pasta sauce with only vegetables in it, is bound to be a poorer eating choice than a product with fewer ingredients.

When the word 'clean' is used to describe food, it basically means the food is as natural and close to nature as possible and free of chemicals and additives as well as antibiotics and hormones if it is an animal form of food. Therefore the 'cleaner' and less processed your food is, the more likely it will provide the nutrients you need for a healthy brain. It is important to read labels because the aim of most food manufacturers is to prolong the shelf-life of the product to maximize profit. They do this by adding additives to their foods and using unscrupulous marketing techniques to sell products to unsuspecting customers. An example of this is stating that certain foods are 'fortified' with specific nutrients without explaining that the nutrients were initially removed in the manufacturing process. Unfortunately, the names listed on processed food labels are also unrecognizable to many people, nor does the fact that they're listed mean they're necessarily safe to consume. Reading food labels gives you the power of choosing foods that support your mental and physical health. As a general rule, foods that are found in the centre of a store are processed foods and will not lead to you feeling light or bright on any level!

Are additives safe?

The levels of what constitutes safe quantities of additives were set many years ago when safety issues were not as well understood and when only a small percentage of available foods contained additives. Today, there are many more additives being added to food than ever before and there is a real risk of interactions between additives, which raises questions about the safety of the amount of additives that are being consumed. Furthermore, as most of these additives are synthetic compounds, we don't have results on what the long-term consequences of consuming large amounts of additives are. The GRAS standard (Generally Regarded As Safe) is applied to the additives that we are consuming. Unfortunately, these additives are tested separately on laboratory animals and not combined. In combination, some of these additives have been found to be very damaging to the brain.

Most processed foods have had their naturally occurring fibre, nutrients and enzymes removed. The consumption of these processed foods results in chemical imbalances in the brain and body with accompanying digestive difficulties. This chemical imbalance also leads to behaviour challenges and malnutrition. Many of these effects are not easily diagnosed and often only manifest later in life. The following table lists the range of additives used in foods.

Additive	Use in foods
Acidity regulators, acids and alkalis	Added to processed foods to influence taste, to stop the growth of some micro-organisms or to influence how other substances in the food function.
Anti-caking agents	Give food a consistent texture and prevent clumping. Help food to flow when poured, such as seasonings.
Anti-foaming agents	Prevent a food or drink from excessive effervescence or foaming when served.
Anti-oxidants	Stop food from spoiling, especially food prone to damage through exposure to oxygen, such as oils.

Additive	Use in foods
Bleaching agents	Used to whiten grains (such as white flour) or to remove the natural pigments in foods.
Bulking agents	Used to make up the volume of a processed food without adding to its energy or calorie count. It's also used when a manufacturer wants to use a cheaper substance than what the food is made of and to replace sugar in low-sugar foods.
Carriers and carrier solvents	Used to change a food additive without changing its original function to make it easier to use or handle. Dissolving, dispersing or diluting the additive can do this.
Colourings	Used to restore or add colour to foods to make them more appealing. This is especially the case in children's processed foods, as children are attracted to bright, unusual colours.
Emulsifiers	Used to ensure the oil and water in the food do not separate into different layers. Margarine uses emulsifiers so that there isn't a layer of fat on the top of the product.
Firming agents or stabilizers	Ensures the different substances in the food remain stable and combined in a consistent manner so that the end-product is uniform in texture and taste, whether it is a solid or semi-solid food.
Flavour enhancers	Improves or enhances the taste and odour of a food. This is again very useful for children's food.
Foaming agents	Used to ensure the gases in foods that need to be aerated stay uniformly distributed through the food. A good example is whipped cream in a can.
Gelling agents	Changes the texture of a food so that it is smooth and gel-like.
Glazing agents	Used to give a coating to the outside of food so it looks shiny or glossy. It is often used on fruit to make it appealing.
Humectants	Added to processed foods to stop them from drying out.
Minerals	These are added when the food's natural mineral content is destroyed during the manufacturing process. Consumers are also led to believe that the food is more nutritious because it has the mineral added.

feed
your
brain

Additive	Use in foods
Preservatives	Added to ensure a food doesn't spoil due to bacteria or micro-organisms.
Propellants	These are pressurized gases added to food to help it expel from its container.
Raising agents	Used to increase the volume of a food by liberating the gases in the food. They are often used in baked goods. Baking powder is a raising agent.
Sweeteners	Used as a cheaper alternative to real sugar to add sweetness to a food without adding to its calorie content. Often added to 'diet' foods and drinks which have their own serious hazards.
Thickeners	Used to thicken food that would otherwise have a different consistency.
Vegetable gums	Used to improve the texture of processed foods as well as to maintain a uniform consistency in the mixture.
Vitamins	Added to foods so the manufacturer can say the food is good for you. Sometimes the vitamin is required in the production process (such as an anti-oxidant). Many foods are now fortified with vitamins, however if the food hadn't been over-processed in the first place, adding the vitamin wouldn't be necessary!
Waxes	Used to make fruit and vegetables look more shiny and appealing. Waxes are made from petrochemicals.

Specific problems caused by specific additives

Most additives are synthetic compounds. We don't have any information on what the long-term consequences of consuming such large amounts of additives are but many are known to cause respiratory tract problems such as asthma, rhinitis and hay fever and skin problems such as hives. Headaches and nausea are other known reactions.

Always check a product's label for additives before buying it. Following are the additives you should avoid because they are particularly harmful to your health, especially when they are combined in a food. Eating unprocessed foods means you don't have to read as many labels!

Tartrazine (102), which is used in soft drinks and orange-coloured snacks, has been implicated in hyperactivity disorder in children. It is termed an anti-nutrient by some researchers as it leaches zinc out of the body, a mineral required for proper neurological functioning as well as growth.

Monosodium glutamate or MSG (621) has been linked to seizures, dizziness, chest pains, nausea, tightness of the face and headaches, diarrhoea and stomach cramps. MSG provides a continuous stimulation of the taste bud receptors, which increases the potential for experiencing the variety of flavours added to the foods. As a result, other foods without this additive begin to taste boring and bland, which is what the food manufacturers want you to experience so that you purchase more of their chemically laden foods. MSG is also called an excitotoxin because it causes specific neurons to become overstimulated. They become incapable of switching off and end up dying.

MSG is a very widely used flavour enhancer and is often put as hydrolysed vegetable protein (HVP) on food labels by manufacturers who know that many people are aware of its negative side effects. HVP is actually made from the brown sludge that is formed on top of vegetables that have been boiled and treated with caustic soda. This brown sludge is scraped off, dried and then sold to food manufacturers to 'enhance' their food products. Unfortunately, the words 'natural flavouring' on a food label does not mean it does not contain MSG. In fact, 20–60 per cent of this additive may contain MSG.

Many artificial flavours cause health issues. Artificial flavours are generally used in concentrations ten times stronger than artificial colours. They also have no numbers on processed food labels, so you can't even check for them. They seem to stop the synthesis of specific detoxifying enzymes, which means that any food with toxic effects can't be broken down and eliminated from the body. This may cause damage to cells and therefore interfere with normal cellular function.

Umami

For thousands of years Japanese cooks have used a special type of seaweed called kombu (*Laminaria japonica*) to enhance the flavour of their foods. When the specific chemical in kombu was first isolated, MSG came into being, leading to a multimillion-dollar food industry. Japanese soldiers during World War II had MSG added to their rations, highlighting the tastelessness of the Americans' rations. This is one of the reasons why Americans embraced the introduction of MSG in the late 1940s. We now know that the specific taste experience that MSG elicits is called 'umami' — the fifth taste after bitter, sour, salty and sweet. When translated, umami means 'deliciousness'. Naturally occurring MSG which is found in tomatoes, mushrooms and kombu seaweed, for example, does not contain the commercially prepared and concentrated form of MSG. Naturally occurring MSG enters the bloodstream slowly during digestion and is therefore not toxic.

In 2006, researchers uncovered a frightening fact: some additives in combination affect brain development. These additives, mainly artificial colours, came to the attention of the public in the United Kingdom when their combined action on neurons was analyzed in a laboratory setting. Brilliant Blue (133), monosodium glutamate (621), Quinoline Yellow (104) and Aspartame (951) in combination stopped the normal growth of neurons and interfered with the signals between neurons. This was one of the first times that an independent research team had looked at the combined effect of additives. Furthermore, the development of neurons was found to be hampered by the amount of additives that would theoretically be consumed in a typical snack and drink. In other words, a typical snack eaten by a child on a regular basis could contain enough of these additives to stop optimal neuronal growth and development.

Assuming that adults would not be affected is short-sighted. We also have the capacity to grow new neurons, which may be hampered by these additives. Unfortunately, no similar research has been done on adults, but erring on the side of caution, I believe it is best to avoid them regardless of your age.

Since then, six other additives have been added to the 'may have an adverse effect on activity and attention in children' list in the United Kingdom: Sunset Yellow (110), Carmoisine (122), Allura Red (129), Tartrazine (102) and Ponceau 4R (124), and sodium benzoate (211). Many of these additives have been banned in countries throughout the world.

It is important to keep in mind that additives can have cumulative effects. They can accumulate in the body, reaching levels of toxicity that have not been tested for, and they can act with other additives, which will increase their effects on the body and brain.

Aspartame

Aspartame requires a special mention as it is made up of three different substances, namely aspartic acid, phenylalanine and methanol (wood alcohol). These substances are released into the bloodstream when aspartame is ingested and the effects of phenylalanine and tyrosine (both amino acids) are increased n humans. High levels of these amino acids in the brain can negatively affect the synthesis of neurotransmitters and bodily functions that are controlled by the autonomic nervous system, such as blood pressure. Aspartame also inhibits the release of glucose into the bloodstream and may reduce the release of serotonin within the brain. Low levels cf serotonin may negatively affect hunger and sleep. Research regularly links aspartame with memory loss, attention deficit disorder (ADD) and headaches. People with mood disorders also seem to be particularly sensitive to it. And aspartame may actually increase appetite, not subdue it! Interestingly, using artificial sweeteners can save food manufacturers as much as one-third of the cost of a bottle of soda. Is it any wonder they love using them?

feed
your
brain

The following table outlines the worst additives found in many food and beauty products.

Acesulfame K (950t)	Indigotine (132)
Allura Red (129)	Monosodium glutamate (621)
Amaranth (123)	Ponceau 4R (124)
Annatto (160b)	Potassium benzoate (212)
Aspartame (951)	Potassium nitrate (249)
Benzoic acid (210)	Propyl-p-hydroxy-benzoate, propylparaben (216)
Brilliant Black (151)	Quinoline Yellow (104)
Brilliant Blue (133)	Saccharin (954)
Brown HT (155)	Sodium benzoate (211)
Butylated hydroxyanisole (BHA) (320)	Sodium metabisulfite (223)
Calcium benzoate (213)	Sodium sulfite (221)
Calcium sulfite (226)	Stannous chloride (512)
Caramel (150a, 150b, 150c and 150d)	Sulfur dioxide (220)
Carmoisine (122)	Sunset Yellow (110)
Erythrosine (127)	Tartrazine (102)
Fast Green (143)	
Green S (142)	

There are only a few safe additives found in many food and beauty products. These include vitamin A/carotene (160), vitamin B1/riboflavin (101), vitamin B3/niacin (375), vitamin C (300–304), vitamin E/tocopherols (306–309), lecithin (322) and pectin (440).

Heavy metals that harm

Heavy metals such as lead, aluminium, arsenic, mercury, copper and cadmium are used extensively in industrial practices and are found in pesticides, insecticides, electroplating and storage batteries. Your home contains these metals in plumbing, various building materials and paints. Mercury was used in dental fillings, although dentists do use other compounds today, such as composite resin. Mercury was also used in vaccines in the form of thimerosal, as a preservative, although it has been replaced with aluminium. These heavy metals are especially damaging to nerve cells, so avoiding exposure to them is very important for the optimal functioning of your central nervous system, and brain.

Milliners used felt and mercury-based compounds to make hats in the eighteenth and nineteenth centuries. Although the character in Lewis Carroll's *Alice in Wonderland* was not based on a hatter but an eccentric furniture dealer, Lewis would have known about the symptoms that hatters presented with in England at the time. Symptoms such as red cheeks, red nose and lips, muscle weakness, increased sensitivity to light, skin rashes, insomnia and memory challenges are all linked to mercury poisoning. Loss of hair, teeth and nails may also occur.

Cadmium from cigarettes may lead to confusion and aggression, while mercury from pesticides and old dental fillings leads to headaches and memory loss. Aluminium from cookware and water is associated with senility, and copper from water pipes leads to anxiety, insomnia and phobias. Lead from past exhaust fumes, paint and industrial facilities has settled in soil, especially near mining or smelting sites. Lead can find its way into our water supply from contaminated soil and leads to hyperactivity, aggression and a low IQ.

What do heavy metals do to the central nervous system?

As the brain is the most sophisticated organ we possess, any cellular damage is far-reaching and noticeable. Some of the reasons the brain is especially susceptible to heavy metals are as follows. The brain has a high fat content, which can lead to the accumulation of heavy metals in cell membranes. Mercury is especially attracted to the fat-rich neural membranes. High blood flow in the brain naturally exposes neurons to the toxicity of heavy metals. Heavy metals also produce free-radical damage in cells, which reduces a cell's ability to function optimally and leads to them being unable to replace themselves effectively. Heavy metals also cause changes in cellular membrane functioning, which in turn negatively influences the way cells absorb and use nutrients and how neurotransmitters communicate with each other. This leads to impairment in learning and development as well as normal cognitive functioning. Cells also become inefficient at expelling toxins when their membranes are damaged.

Because we live in an environment that contains heavy metals, it is important to know how to protect the body against their toxicity and remove them from our cells. Vitamin C, zinc, magnesium, selenium and essential fatty acids (EFAs) all protect against the accumulation of heavy metals due to their ability to keep cell membranes working optimally. Green foods containing chlorophyll allow the body to excrete heavy metals. Sulfur-containing compounds such as garlic, onions, eggs and a supplement called MSM (methylsulfonylmethane) all help to eliminate heavy metals from the body. Apples and citrus fruits contain a compound called pectin, which aids the body in getting rid of heavy metals.

As useful as a detoxifying diet can be, it may not be effective for severe heavy-metal toxicity. If you suspect that you may have been exposed to heavy metals and need to get rid of them, contact a qualified naturopath or nutrition-minded physician who will suggest a program of chelation, whereby heavy metals are ushered out of the body safely. Furthermore, mercury fillings should be avoided at all costs as they provide ongoing poisoning. If you have this type of fillings, then discuss their removal with a dentist experienced in removing them. See page 263 for further resources.

Common chemicals to avoid

More than 3000 chemicals are produced by various industries but only about twelve have been adequately tested for their effects on the brain. Unfortunately, many of these chemicals are commonly encountered in the average home and could easily be avoided when people are made aware of their dangers. Researchers now know that many chemicals negatively impact learning, attention, memory, social behaviour and IQ. Many of these compounds are called persistent organic pollutants (POPs) because they accumulate in the natural environment and may take hundreds of years to break down. The following table highlights the common chemicals used in many household goods and products. All should be avoided.

Chemical	Use in industry
Phthalates (also called plasticizers)	This group of chemicals gives products flexibility. They are found in the lining of metallic food containers, children's toys, shower curtains, flooring, adhesives, tubing, PVC window frames, detergents, paints and plastic wrap. Unfortunately, they are also found in shampoos, gels, hair sprays, sunscreen, perfume and powder. They find their way into foods such as fish, eggs, dairy and breast milk. They are absorbed through skin or inhaled, and are stored in fat cells. Increased allergies have been linked to this chemical.
Dioxins (or PCDDs)	A by-product of the manufacture of substances such as PVC, metal smelting, bleaching of paper and some natural environmental events such as forest fires and volcanoes. They are POPs and present in dietary sources of fat as they accumulate in the fatty tissues of the animals we eat and then become stored in our fat cells. They are responsible for hormonal dysfunction, central nervous system problems, thyroid disorders, immune dysfunction, as well insulin insens tivity which leads to diabetes.
PCBs	A group of chemicals which were used as stabilizers in PVC coatings of electrical wiring, plasticizers in cements and various paints, pesticide extenders and wood floor finishes. They were banned in the USA in the 1970s due to their toxicity, however they are still used in some countries. They still form part of our ecosystem as they are long-lived and don't break down naturally. They are similar to dioxins in their structure and their toxic activity on the human body and wildlife. They also accumulate in fat. These dangerous toxins cause skin reactions, liver dysfunction, fatigue, hormonal imbalance through endocrine disruption, and may be involved in central nervous system dysfunction.
PFOA (Perfluorooctanoic acid or C8)	Used by industry to make fluoropolymers, which provide non-stick surfaces on cookware and waterproof clothing. Products known as Teflon® may have trace amounts of this chemical. Birth defects have been linked to this chemical among workers who are exposed to Teflon chemicals. Research is still underway to determine whether people who use it regularly in their homes are in danger too.

Chemical	Use in industry
Carbamates	These are used in fungicides, insecticides, anti-parasitic treatments, wood treatments and as a component of synthetic rubber. They are also used as growth-promoters on animal farms because they slow down the metabolic rate of the animals, increasing their bulk. Consequently, they are also found in many drink and food products, some medicines and treated wood. They have been found to cause damage to the brain and impair the energy-production process.
Solvents	Chemicals used extensively in many products we think of as 'natural' to our daily lives such as polystyrene, dry-cleaning chemicals, detergents, toiletries, synthetic fragrances, solvents for paint, shoe creams, synthetic rubbers, sealants for metal foil covers, foods in polystyrene containers and exhaust fumes. Exposure to solvents over time can lead to brain and nerve damage, which can lead to learning disorders as well as visual and hearing impairments.
BPA (Bisphenol A)	A synthetic compound used to make plastics and often found in the lining of tin cans. It is thought to mimic estrogen, which means that it may pose serious threats to a developing (and adult) hormonal system.
Pesticides	Commonly used to kill bugs and pests on soil-grown foods. These compounds work by destroying the brain and nervous system of insects by interfering in the transmission of their nerve impulses — they do this to humans and animals too. It is important to mention here that meat contains about fourteen times more pesticides than plant foods, and dairy products have five and a half times more. Animal-origin foods have concentrated amounts of chemicals in them simply because they are at the top of the food chain. When you choose to eat more plant-based foods, you are choosing to eat foods that are less contaminated with chemicals and therefore better for your brain.
Synthetic fragrances	Synthetic fragrances have no benefit apart from imparting a pleasant smell. We don't know what else they are giving us because we breathe them in and our skin absorbs them. Natural fragrances, which come from essential plant extracts, offer extra benefits such as antibacterial and antiviral properties, as well as healing and protection for skin.
Fluoride	This chemical has been shown to be neurotoxic in animal models and may cause neuorotoxicity in adults with acute doses. Recent research investigating whether children can suffer from excess fluoride exposure has yielded frightening results: children in high fluoride areas had significantly lower IQ scores than children who live in low fluoride areas.

Your hard-working liver

Although the liver has many important functions to perform in the body, its main role is to filter the blood that comes from the digestive tract before it moves into the rest of the body and brain. This means that it has to filter out any toxins that could potentially cause harm, and detoxify chemicals that you've ingested. It also has to metabolize any ingested drugs. Obviously, when your body is exposed to heavy metals, the liver has to step up and try to get rid of them. It has three primary ways of doing this: the Phase I, Phase II and Phase III liver detoxification pathways. A healthy liver is very important for brain function because 60 per cent of the amino acids we require for optimal functioning, many of which get converted into neurotransmitters, are produced by the liver.

During Phase I, the liver is focusing on transforming the damaging compounds into a different form, using specific enzymes, so as to make them ready for the next stage of detoxification. The liver needs iron, vitamins B2, B3, B6 and B12 as well as folate and various amino acids to perform this task. These compounds are often even more toxic than the original compounds, so they need to be moved into Phase II quickly and efficiently. During Phase II, the liver again needs vitamins B6, B12 and folate as well as the amino acids glycine, glutamate, cysteine, methionine, taurine and the potent anti-oxidant glutathione to transform the compounds of Phase I into a less toxic form. During Phase III the focus is on moving the toxins out of the liver to the kidneys and the digestive tract. Glutathione is again necessary during this phase as is plenty of water and fibre.

Organic is best

When purchasing fruit and vegetables remember that the pesticides and insecticides used on conventional produce act as nerve agents on the bugs and have been linked to neurodevelopmental problems in humans. Choosing organic produce (including organic meat and wild-caught fish) whenever possible is just basic protection for your brain.

It isn't possible to avoid all the hazardous chemicals and toxins that are now part of life on Earth but there are a few simple ways to help your body to detox naturally on a daily basis:

1. Ensure that you are drinking enough pure, clean water.

2. Ensure that your food choices contain enough fibre to keep your digestive tract working efficiently.

3. If consuming meat make sure that it is not charred during cooking. Stewed or slow-cooked meat is easier to digest.

4. Limit or, better still, eliminate the use of synthetic materials in the home, such as conventional paints or carpets.

5. Limit your intake of over-the-counter medications, which cause extra stress on your liver. Always discuss with your medical practitioner any changes you may want to make with your medication.

6. Use ceramic-coated cookware instead of conventional non-stick products.

Action plan

Five things you can do to remove additives from your diet AND reduce exposure to dangerous environmental toxins are:

1. Replace your favourite, additive-filled snack with a healthier alternative.

2. Whatever tomato sauce or soya sauce you use, replace it with a healthier and additive-free option. Replace any canned foods that have preservatives, flavourings or other additives with another variety that has none. Make sure the cans do not contain BPA. Check that the variety of bread or crackers you consume is free of additives.

3. Choose organic foods where possible and start growing your own lettuces and herbs in your back garden or balcony.

4. Do not reheat food in plastic containers.

5. Check that both your household cleaning products and body products, such as toothpaste, shampoos, deodorants and skin moisturizers are free of fragrances and other toxic chemicals. Buy certified organic if possible.

See the Resources section for more supportive information.

CHAPTER 4

The vitamins and minerals your brain needs

Health food stores are packed with bottles of vitamins and minerals, as well as a variety of other mixtures, promising to increase energy, reduce ageing and provide us with the missing nutrients that processed foods lack. Unfortunately, many people do not know exactly why we need vitamins and minerals nor how to supplement with them wisely. A lack of these nutrients can result in very poor health, with the brain being especially sensitive to deficiencies in specific vitamins and minerals. Supplementing your diet with the right nutrients can lead to huge improvements in health generally, and a great boost to mental wellbeing.

The aim of this chapter is to explain the role of vitamins and minerals in brain health specifically and to highlight which ones are especially important. Supplementation may be necessary at times to improve brain health.

What do vitamins and minerals actually do?

A vitamin is an organic substance that is essential to life — essential because it has to be obtained via your diet because your body can't make it. Vitamins are contained in food and need to be converted into various components to sustain life.

A mineral is an inorganic substance that is also essential to life. Minerals need to be obtained from the food we eat because without them, vitamins couldn't be used properly and we couldn't function optimally. In the past few decades we have discovered how important minerals are for brain function and what happens when the brain is deficient in them.

Vitamins and minerals are responsible for turning glucose into energy and helping to convert amino acids into messenger neurotransmitters, basic fats into specialized fats, and choline and serine into phospholipids. They help with the building and rebuilding of the brain (and body), which occurs continuously, and to keep the whole central nervous system running smoothly. When they are in short supply, the efficient running of all your cells is influenced negatively.

What is malnutrition?

When people think of malnutrition, they generally think of an emaciated body: a thin and frail skeletal frame. Unfortunately, this definition is no longer correct. Malnutrition is either caused by a lack of the correct nutrients, an imbalance of nutrients, or an excess of particular nutrients. This means that too much of the wrong kinds of nutrients still leaves a body malnourished, even if it is overweight or obese. A new classification for this type of malnutrition is called multiple micronutrient depletion or 'Type B malnutrition'. This condition can also be called 'over nutrition'. Obviously, this state of nutrition does not support balanced mood, clear thinking and emotional poise!

Marginal vitamin 'deficiency'

A marginal vitamin deficiency is the 'no-man's land' between adequate nutrient status and the point when physical symptoms of deficiencies present. A precise definition of a marginal vitamin deficiency, from the book *Smart Food* by Arthur and Ruth Winter, is 'a state of gradual vitamin depletion in which there is evidence of personal lack of wellbeing associated with impairment of certain biochemical reactions, that depend on sufficient amounts of vitamin.'

Marginal deficiencies are not easy to identify, however there are researchers who now believe that vague psychological symptoms may be a clue to this grey area. The traditional view held that if a person didn't show the clinical signs of classic deficiency diseases such as scurvy, beriberi, rickets or pellagra, then they were adequately nourished. Now we know that the ability to detect and treat a disease at the earliest stages of development is extremely beneficial to a positive outcome. Therefore, it would be very useful to be able to detect a marginal deficiency before symptoms appeared.

Vitamin deficiency doesn't appear overnight. Micronutrient body stores gradually deplete. It is only when marked behavioural and personality changes such as depression, anxiety, irritability, insomnia and loss of appetite appear that a vitamin deficiency is apparent. If depletion continues, death will occur. Although classical deficiency diseases have all but disappeared in most modern, First World countries, marginal deficiencies may very well be increasing due to nutrient-deficient diets. They are more subtle and difficult to identify, although research in recent years has highlighted a number of psychological symptoms that may be useful in assessing whether marginal deficiencies are present. Fortunately, today we also have biochemical analysis to assist in determining the nutrient status of a body via blood, plasma or urine samples. Another method used is to assess a substance or process that is dependent on the vitamin's presence. If the vitamin isn't present, the substance or process will be influenced negatively, highlighting its absence.

In studies done on human starvation, a lack of thiamin presented itself with feelings of anxiety, hysteria, nausea, depression and lack of appetite. A general lack of wellbeing was also noted. These symptoms preceded the clinical stage of beriberi. And once thiamin was added to the diet of these subjects, these psychological symptoms disappeared within a short period of time. Other studies, under carefully controlled laboratory conditions, induced deficiencies of vitamin C, thiamin and riboflavin (vitamin B2) in human subjects. They were then given a personality test. Scores indicated that depression, hysteria, hypochondria and even psychopathic tendencies were linked to these marginal states of deficiency. These symptoms appeared before any physical signs of deficiency appeared.

It is therefore entirely possible that millions of people are living with marginal deficiencies, severely impacting their quality of life. Adequate brain function is not *optimal* brain function and many researchers are now of the opinion that substantial segments of the population are not obtaining the levels of vitamins and minerals needed for optimal brain function. Although marginal deficiencies in minerals are not as well documented, a deficiency in the minerals magnesium and zinc is implicated in depression, anxiety, eating disorders and psychiatric disorders.

Which vitamins do what?

Various nutrients have been shown to facilitate the production of energy within the brain's mitochondria, as well as support other functions within cells that in turn influence cognitive function. Water-soluble vitamins are hard to overdose on, unless you take them in excess. Fat-soluble vitamins on the other hand are easier to overdose on, however this is not a concern if supplements are used in the correct quantities. The brain needs both of these types of vitamins.

The reason the following list of vitamins and minerals only includes 'best plant sources' is because most people don't eat enough plant foods. By including more of these plant sources of vitamins and minerals in your diet, you will be adding not only the vitamins and minerals mentioned but also phytonutrients, which are extremely important for optimal cognitive health.

B group vitamins

B vitamins are necessary for neural activity. They turn glucose into energy, are co-factors for making neurotransmitters, help to transport oxygen and help protect the brain from toxins and oxidants. A proper balance of these vitamins must be maintained to gain maximum benefits from them. The brain, to convert glucose to energy, uses up the B vitamins very quickly, so it is best that they are replenished regularly during the day through snacks and meals, and with a supplement in the morning, if required.

VITAMIN B1

Vitamin B1, or thiamin, is an essential nutrient and is only stored in small quantities by the body, so regular supplies are crucial to brain function. An inability to concentrate, poor memory, irritability and confused thinking are some of the symptoms of a thiamin-deficient diet. Severe deficiencies lead to brain damage. Recent research has yielded dramatic and pleasing results with many behavioural challenges such as hyperactivity, learning difficulties, tantrums and anxiety being reduced by multivitamin (including thiamin) supplements. Extreme signs of thiamin deficiency are tender muscles, stomach pains, constipation, tingling hands, depression, nervous disorders, loss of memory and rapid heartbeat.

The best plant sources of thiamin are wholegrain cereals, nuts, watercress, capsicum (bell peppers), lettuce, zucchini (courgette), asparagus, mushrooms, peas, cabbage, potatoes and pulses (legumes).

VITAMIN B2

Vitamin B2, or riboflavin, is an essential nutrient required for energy production, converting fats, sugars and protein into energy and regulating body acidity. It is also important for hair, nails, skin, eyes and tissue repair. Extreme signs of deficiency are lack of energy, numbness, burning and itchy eyes, light sensitivity, sore tongue, dull hair, and dry cracked lips.

The best plant sources of vitamin B2 are almonds, pumpkin seeds (pepitas), bean sprouts, mushrooms, cabbage, watercress, asparagus, broccoli, pumpkin and tomatoes.

VITAMIN B3

Vitamin B3, or niacin, is an essential nutrient and one of the primary boosters of energy production in the mitochondria. It therefore has a special place in protecting the brain and boosting memory because when energy runs low, brain cells function less effectively. It is also essential for a healthy digestive system, circulation and skin and is needed for balancing blood sugar. Extreme signs of deficiency include a lack of energy, insomnia, headaches, memory challenges, scaly skin, bleeding, sore gums, anxiety and depression.

The best plant sources of niacin are cabbage, asparagus, tomatoes, cauliflower, zucchini (courgette), squash, pulses (legumes), potatoes, peas, peanuts, sunflower seeds, tahini, pine nuts (pine kernels), mushrooms, green leafy vegetables, prunes and figs.

VITAMIN B5

Vitamin B5, or pantothenic acid, is an essential nutrient and helps to improve memory and mental alertness. It is essential for energy production and brain and nerve function. It also controls fat metabolism and maintains healthy hair and skin. Extreme signs of deficiency include lack of energy, teeth grinding, muscle cramps or tremors, poor concentration, nausea or vomiting and burning feet or tender heels.

The best plant sources of vitamin B5 are alfalfa sprouts, mushrooms, watercress, tomatoes, broccoli, cabbage, whole-wheat (wholemeal) bread, celery, strawberries, avocados, lentils, peas and squash.

VITAMIN B6

Vitamin B6, or pyridoxine, is an essential nutrient. Deficiencies are linked to suboptimal brain performance and concentration and memory difficulties. This vitamin is very important because it is required to synthesize neurotransmitters. It is also necessary for converting amino acids into serotonin — a deficiency that can lead to depression and other mental disturbances. Vitamin B6 is essential for assimilating fat and protein, to produce healthy red blood cells and for normal brain function and hormone production. It is a natural antidepressant and diuretic and helps to control allergic reactions and maintain a healthy immune system. Extreme signs of deficiency are dermatitis, depression, poor dream recall, water retention, irritability, flaky skin, lack of energy, tingling hands and anaemia. Anxiety and depression are also symptoms of B6 deficiency.

The best plant sources of vitamin B6 are capsicum (bell peppers), lentils, red kidney beans, onions, seeds, asparagus, watercress, bananas, nuts and cruciferous vegetables such as cabbage, cauliflower and broccoli.

Pyroluria or 'mauve factor'

Pyroluria (also known as pyrrole disorder or hemepyrrole) is a metabolic condition where a key component of haemoglobin (kryptopyrrole or KP) is overproduced by the liver. It is also sometimes called 'mauve factor' as it turns the testing paper mauve, or pale purple, when kryptopyrroles are found in urine samples of sufferers. Although it is a genetically determined condition, severe stress and/or trauma at a young age and chronic infection before adulthood, as well as heavy metal toxicity, have been linked to the onset of pyroluria. Stress and age contribute to its severity. In this condition excess kryptopyrrole binds to vitamin B6 as well as zinc depleting the body of these two important nutrients, which act as co-factors in a multitude of enzyme reactions required for optimal mental and physical health. The essential fatty acid, omega-6, is also depleted in this condition. Symptoms of vitamin B6 and zinc deficiency include anxiety, mood instability, anger, memory challenges, depression and poor stress control. A very pale skin and an inability to get tanned as well as abnormal fat distribution, poor dream recall and sensitivity to light and sound are also signs that pyroluria may be present. Ongoing stress worsens the symptoms considerably. A urine test measures the level of krytopyrroles and determines the presence of this disorder and its severity. Women are more prone to developing this disorder than men. See a qualified naturopath or a nutrition-minded physician if you suspect you have pyroluria.

VITAMIN B12

Vitamin B12, or cyanocobalamin, is an essential nutrient critically important for optimal brain function. Cyanocobalamin needs to be converted into methylcobalamin before it can be used. If you have a polymorphism on the MTHFR gene, then you may not be as capable of converting it into this usable form. See page 112 for more information about the MTHFR gene. A deficiency can lead to neurological damage, disorientation, memory challenges and dementia. Cyanocobalamin is essential for the formation of red blood cells, the synthesis of deoxyribonucleic acid (DNA), to maintain a healthy nervous system and to increase energy levels. It also has a role to play in axon myelination, which is critically important for neuronal messaging. It also protects neurons from degeneration. Vegans (people who consume no animal products) and vegetarians do need to supplement with this important vitamin, as it is not present in plant foods. Vegans must use B12-fortified yeast products, B12-fortified breakfast cereals or a B12 supplement. You will need to supplement with methyl-B12 if you have a polymorphism on the MTHFR gene and cannot convert cyanocobalamin to methyl-cobalamin efficiently.

Extreme signs of deficiency include an increased risk of infection, fatigue, poor hair condition, eczema or dermatitis, nervous complaints, mouth oversensitive to temperature, constipation and anaemia.

Can B-vitamin deficiencies be confused with mental disorders?

The similarities between the symptoms of B-vitamin deficiencies and neuropsychiatric disorders are eerily similar. In fact, as you will see in the table below, many of them are exactly the same.

B-vitamin deficiency symptoms	Neuropsychiatric disorder symptoms
Anxiety	Severe anxiety
Fatigue	Severe fatigue
Depression	Depression
Paranoia	Paranoia
Confusion	Confusion
Hostility and/or rage	Anger and/or aggression, accompanied by suicidal thoughts/tendencies
Fears	Morbid fears

Unfortunately, only enlightened physicians will request a B-vitamin test before they prescribe anxiolytics, antidepressants or other anti-psychotic medications.

Checking to see if you are deficient in B vitamins is very simple. A simple pinprick will produce a drop of blood that a laboratory will use to assess your homocysteine level. High levels of homocysteine are an indication of low levels of B vitamins, especially vitamin B6, B12 and folic acid.

In addition, have yourself tested for the MTHFR polymorphism (see page 112 for more information) as you may need specifically tailored supplements.

The anti-oxidant trio

Most people are exposed to toxins on a daily basis via air pollution and various household and body products. Stress adds to this onslaught. Free radicals, the unstable compounds produced in the body and brain from these toxins, can wreak havoc on essential fats, phospholipids and proteins. Fortunately, if your diet contains enough anti-oxidants, they will be able to provide the antidote to many of these damaging free radicals.

The most important vitamins required for brain function are vitamin E (a fat-soluble vitamin), vitamin C and beta-carotene, which is the precursor to vitamin A (also fat soluble). Other anti-oxidants that aid brain function include selenium, glutathione, anthocyanins (found in berries), lipoic acid and co-enzyme Q10. Burnt food introduces damaging free radicals to the body, so be sure to cook food carefully.

VITAMIN A

Vitamin A (found in beta-carotene in plants and retinol in animals) is an essential nutrient and critical for vision, bone growth, skin and tissue repair, as well as building healthy cells in the gut and brain. It acts as an anti-oxidant and protects the immune system. Vitamin A-rich foods don't mind being heated, but it is better to steam root vegetables lightly to retain some enzymes instead of overcooking them.

The eyes are part of the brain and need the right fats, as well as vitamin A to function optimally. Extreme signs of deficiency are poor night vision, mouth ulcers, acne, thrush or cystitis, dry skin, diarrhoea and a lowered resistance to infection — especially respiratory disorders.

The best plant sources of vitamin A are sweet potatoes, carrots, apricots, melon, asparagus, tangerines, capsicum (bell peppers), broccoli, squash, mango, watercress, papayas, pumpkin, tomatoes and green leafy vegetables (such as kale, spinach, Brussels sprouts and collard greens).

VITAMIN C

Vitamin C, or ascorbic acid, is an essential nutrient and a very strong anti-oxidant that readily passes through the blood–brain barrier. It is concentrated in very high levels in the adrenal glands and brain tissue (almost fifteen times higher than in other areas of the body). It contributes to the creation of neurotransmitters and protects cells from free radical damage. It also facilitates the transmission of messages throughout the brain and can directly influence electrical impulses. It is therefore a primary player in determining the quantity and quality of brain transmissions.

Extreme signs of deficiency include a lack of energy, low immunity, bleeding or tender gums, nosebleeds, slow wound healing, easy bruising and red pimples on skin. The best plant sources of vitamin C are citrus fruits, melons, tomatoes, capsicum (bell peppers), potatoes, broccoli, strawberries, watercress, cabbage, peas and kiwi fruit. Vitamin C is destroyed by heat, so it's best not to heat these foods.

VITAMIN E

Vitamin E or tocopherol is an essential nutrient and required to keep your brain functioning optimally. As the brain is mostly fat, it is highly susceptible to fat-spoiling free radicals. Vitamin E, in adequate quantities, ensures the destruction of free radicals, thereby ensuring the swift and accurate transmission of messages in the brain.

Extreme signs of deficiency are slow wound healing, loss of muscle tone, easy bruising and exhaustion after light exercise. It is best to use vitamin E-containing oils without heating them, as this causes damage to the delicate fatty acids.

The best plant sources are seeds, nuts, cold-pressed vegetable oils, wholegrain products, beans, peas, sweet potatoes (kumera), oats, cereals and green leafy vegetables.

The power of anti-oxidants

Without oxygen we cannot live — it is the basis of all life on this planet. Every cell in the human body needs oxygen. Without it, we can't release the energy from our food that facilitates all our body processes, including the complicated workings of our energy-hungry brains. Oxygen, being very reactive, loses an electron in the process of being broken down for energy and becomes an unstable molecule. These unstable molecules then search for a healthy cell's stable molecule to pair with, so that they can be stable again. In the process they end up creating more dangerous, unstable molecules or what are called free radicals.

The mitochondria, the energy producers in our cells, become less effective as we age because they produce more free radicals and, in turn, become more damaged by the free radicals themselves. It's a catch-22 situation — the mitochondria work harder for less energy, become increasingly ineffective and produce substances that damage themselves! Anti-oxidants neutralize these damaging free radicals by acting as electron donors to de-activate these 'bad' molecules and thus prevent them from harming healthy cells. Anti-oxidants also reduce and prevent the production of these free radicals. Therefore, the more foods rich in anti-oxidants you eat, the healthier you'll be because there will be more anti-oxidants to mop up the free radicals that are being produced naturally in your body and brain. And remember, the brain is the most metabolically active organ in the body so it is producing many more free radicals. Anti-oxidants will also help deal with the extra load of anti-nutrients that you come into contact with in this modern, polluted world.

Other important vitamins

VITAMIN D

Vitamin D, or calciferol, is an essential nutrient made up of two components: D2 (known as ergocalciferol) and D3 (cholecalciferol). This compound can be synthesized by the body when it is exposed to sunlight, which means that it's not technically a vitamin and has been called a hormone instead. However, it is essential for the formation of healthy bones and teeth, as well as helping the body to absorb and retain calcium and phosphorous. It also has a stimulating effect on specific substances in the brain called neurotrophins, which regulate neuronal cells. Research into its effects on cognitive function has highlighted that low levels of vitamin D are related to low mood and impairment in cognitive function.

The best plant source of vitamin D is cold-pressed vegetable oil. The action of sunlight on the skin also produces vitamin D, and as many people now avoid the sun because of its potentially damaging effects, many people are deficient in this essential nutrient. If you live in the Northern Hemisphere, you may need to take a vitamin D supplement. Getting one to two hours of sun exposure every day, in the early morning or late afternoon, to avoid skin damage, is a good way to get adequate amounts of this important compound, as well as eating foods that are high in vitamin D. Foods that are rich in vitamin D include eggs, butter and fish, which contains the highest amount of this nutrient. It is difficult, if not impossible, to get enough vitamin D from food alone if you are not exposed to sunshine every day. Signs of vitamin D deficiency include muscle weakness or stiffness, backache, hair loss, anaemia and a softening of the bones and teeth. Long-term deficiency in children results in rickets, and recent research indicates that a deficiency may also be linked to adolescent obesity, although this may be linked to a lack of sunshine AND a lack of exercise.

VITAMIN K

Vitamin K is an essential nutrient and required for controlling blood clotting, bone formation and heart health. It is a fat-soluble vitamin.

Vitamin K is found in three forms: K1 (phylloquinone), K2 (menaquinone) and a synthetic form, K3 (menadione), which is best avoided. Vitamin K1 is found primarily in plants such as lettuce, cabbage, cauliflower, beans, broccoli, peas, watercress, asparagus, potatoes and tomatoes, as well as in fermented foods such as miso. Vitamin K2 is produced by the good bacteria that inhabit your digestive tract, although you may need to supplement with a probiotic if your digestive health isn't optimal — see page 50. Increasing your intake of fermented foods will naturally improve your K2 levels. K2 is also found in animal products such as butter, soft and hard cheese and meat.

Extreme signs of vitamin K deficiency are poor blood clotting, regular and copious nose bleeding and bone formation problems.

FOLATE OR VITAMIN B9

Folate, or vitamin B9, is the name used for a group of specific vitamins. They are essential nutrients required for oxygen delivery to the brain, proper cell division and the formation of red blood cells. They also enhance the plasma concentrations of the fatty acids DHA and EPA, which are essential for brain and nerve function. A lack of folate has been linked to many psychiatric disorders, as well as subtle cognitive difficulties, such as changes in mood and memory challenges. The different forms of folate are:

- Folic acid: a synthetic compound used in certain processed foods and supplements. The enzyme required to process folic acid in the liver and make it usable may not be active enough to break it all down. Excess folic acid may also mask a deficiency in vitamin B12, a critically important nutrient required for optimal central nervous system functioning.

- Folinic acid: a compound that has been partly metabolized along the pathway from folic acid to 5-MTHF, the active form of folate. It is found in supplements and may be a better choice than folic acid.

- 5-MTHF (5-methyltetrahydrofolate) is the active form of folate found in specific supplements, which may be helpful for people who have an inability (genetically or otherwise) to break down folic acid efficiently.

- Women planning on becoming pregnant, or who are already pregnant, may need to supplement their diet with either folinic acid or 5-MTHF, as this group of nutrients is critically important for the development of the unborn child's central nervous system. See also page 112 for more information about folic acid and the MTHFR gene.

- Extreme signs of deficiency include appetite loss, anaemia, prematurely greying hair, anxiety, depression, cracked lips, eczema and neural tube defects in babies.

- The best plant sources are nuts, beetroot (beet), parsley, spinach, sprouts, sesame seeds, hazelnuts, cashew nuts, walnuts, broccoli, avocados, whole-wheat (wholemeal) products, asparagus, pulses (legumes) and bananas.

Which minerals do what?

Although minerals are essential, they are not all required in the same quantity. Some are major minerals and needed in larger quantities while others, called trace elements, are minerals required in lesser amounts.

Major minerals

CALCIUM

Calcium is an essential nutrient. It is critically important for the building and maintaining of healthy bones and teeth as well as the smooth running of the nervous system and muscle function. It ensures skin, bone and teeth health and relieves sore muscles. Calcium maintains the correct acid–alkaline balance in the body and promotes a healthy heart. Extreme signs of deficiency include brittle, soft bones and teeth, insomnia, joint pain, arthritis and muscle weakness.

The best plant sources of calcium are green leafy vegetables, parsley, globe artichokes, prunes, sesame seeds, almonds, broccoli, watercress, cabbage, pumpkin seeds (pepitas), pulses (legumes) and dried figs.

MAGNESIUM

Magnesium is an essential nutrient and increases the anti-oxidant power of vitamin E, as well as being a powerful free-radical scavenger on its own. It is an indispensable brain nutrient, boosting memory. It is also involved with maintaining the metabolic viability of neurons. It is the most important micronutrient for the support of healthy nerve and mental function. Magnesium inhibits excessive excitatory activity within the central nervous system, while promoting the release of the inhibitory neurotransmitter, gamma-aminobutyric acid (GABA), which relaxes the mind. It is essential for healthy bones and teeth, as well as normal growth and nerve function. It helps muscles to remain healthy, enabling them to relax — important for the heart muscles and nervous system. It is involved as a co-factor in many enzymes in the body. It is also very important for optimal cognitive development and maintenance, as it helps to regulate the central and peripheral nervous systems.

Some signs of magnesium deficiency are a difficulty handling external stimuli, general irritability, fatigue and poor concentration, as well as sleeping difficulties, short-term memory loss, emotional ups and downs and being easily angered, discouraged or depressed. Being easily startled and sensitive to loud noises and sounds is another sign of a deficiency in this essential mineral.

Extreme signs of deficiency include weak bones and muscles, muscle tremors or spasms, heart palpitations, insomnia, high blood pressure, hyperactivity, loss of appetite, lethargy, constipation, irritability and depression.

The best plant sources of magnesium are almonds, cashew nuts, pecan nuts, Brazil nuts, cooked beans, potato skin, raisins, green peas and garlic. All green leafy vegetables contain magnesium in varying degrees.

POTASSIUM

Potassium is an essential nutrient required for water balance, normal blood pressure and heart functioning. It enables nutrients to move into cells and waste products to move out of cells and helps the secretion of insulin for blood sugar control. It assists with metabolism and stimulates peristalsis.

Extreme signs of deficiency include thirst, fatigue, weakness, mental confusion and raised blood pressure, as well as an irregular, rapid heartbeat, pins and needles, irritability, cellulite, low blood pressure and a swollen abdomen.

The best plant sources are watercress, endive, celery, cabbage, parsley, zucchini (courgette), cauliflower, radishes, pumpkin, mushrooms and bananas.

SODIUM

Sodium is an essential nutrient required for muscle and nerve function and the regulation of body fluids to prevent dehydration. Extreme signs of deficiency include dehydration, muscle weakness, high blood pressure, dizziness, rapid pulse, mental apathy, headache, nausea and cramps.

The best plant sources of sodium are olives, beetroot (beet), celery, cabbage, watercress and red kidney beans.

CHLORIDE

Chloride is an essential nutrient required to regulate the fluid balance in the body. It is also important in keeping digestion working properly by helping to produce hydrochloric acid in the stomach. Deficiencies are rare unless a lot of fluid has been lost, such as in excessive vomiting or diarrhoea or prolonged sweating.

The best sources of chloride are seaweed, sea salt, olives, whole rye and soy sauce.

Trace elements

CHROMIUM

Chromium is an essential nutrient required to maintain stable blood sugar levels by increasing insulin efficiency. This is important as a stable supply of blood glucose is necessary for optimal brain function. Chromium is essential for normalizing hunger and reducing cravings as it forms part of GTF (glucose tolerance factor), which helps to balance blood sugar. Chromium also helps protect DNA and ribonucleic acid (RNA) and is essential for heart health.

Extreme signs of deficiency are addiction to sweet foods, excessive thirst, irritability or dizziness after six hours without food, the need for frequent snacks, cold hands and an excessive desire for sleep or daytime drowsiness.

The best plant sources of chromium are rye bread, potatoes, apples, parsnips, cornmeal and wholegrains, tomatoes, and cos (romaine) lettuce.

COPPER

Copper is an essential nutrient. It is necessary for the growth and development of the brain, heart, connective tissue and bone. The formation of red blood cells as well as the use of and absorption of iron requires copper. It is also involved in the formation of various enzymes. Copper plays a balancing act with zinc because too much copper will reduce zinc stores and vice versa. Excess copper is very damaging to the central nervous system.

Extreme signs of copper deficiency include anaemia, an irregular heartbeat, skin pigment loss and thyroid problems.

The best plant sources of copper are sesame seeds, cashew nuts, soya beans, sunflower seeds, macadamia nuts, lentils, blackstrap molasses, dried fruits, avocado and chickpeas (garbanzo beans).

IODINE

Iodine is an essential nutrient used in the production of hormones released by the thyroid gland. These thyroid hormones are used in every single cell in the human body. Iodine is essential for the normal development of the brain. Exposure to many of the toxins that are now in our environment, as well as diets high in refined carbohydrates, increases the need for iodine. Severe iodine deficiency during pregnancy may cause cretinism in children, a condition of stunted physical growth, mental retardation and speech and hearing impairment.

Iodine's involvement with thyroid function will influence brain development, as the thyroid hormones play a critical role in neurological processes, such as neuronal cell differentiation, migration and maturation, as well as synaptic plasticity and neurotransmission.

Extreme signs of iodine deficiency include sluggish metabolism, apathy, dry skin and hair as well as depression, irritability and difficulty concentrating.

The best plant source of iodine is seaweed.

IRON

Iron is an essential nutrient required for the production of red blood cells. This nutrient is also vital in the process of myelination — the formation of a specialized covering of a neuron's axon with fatty acids and protein. Lack of myelin would therefore adversely affect speed of processing, attention, focus and cognitive activity. Iron is also involved in various neurotransmitter functions and is therefore essential for optimal cognitive function as well as development. It is essential for healthy muscles and blood and transporting oxygen and carbon dioxide to and from cells. It is vital for energy production, being a component of various enzymes.

Lack of iron is common in people with anaemia. The need for iron can increase by 50 per cent during adolescence for both sexes. Unfortunately, if iron deficiency occurs very early in life, the damage may be irreversible and supplementation will not be able to reverse the damage. Lack of iron is also the most common nutrient deficiency in the world, having a negative impact on the intellectual development of those children who are deficient in it.

There are two forms of iron: those attached to a heme protein and those not attached to a heme protein. Plants contain the non-heme form of iron, which is absorbed less efficiently than the heme form found in animal foods. Relying on only non-heme iron from plants may not be sufficient to relieve iron deficiency.

Extreme signs of deficiency include anaemia, a sore, pale tongue, low resistance to infection, loss of appetite, sensitivity to cold, fatigue and listlessness. Iron deficiency has also been linked to lower grades in school as well as symptoms of ADHD.

The best plant sources of iron are pumpkin seeds (pepitas), parsley, almonds and cashew nuts, raisins, Brazil nuts, walnuts, dates, sesame seeds, pecan nuts, green leafy vegetables, prunes, dried apricots, tofu, wholegrains and pulses (legumes).

MANGANESE
Manganese is an essential nutrient required for the formation of healthy bones, tissue, cartilage and nerves. It activates more than twenty enzymes, is important for the production of insulin, stabilizes blood sugar, promotes healthy DNA and RNA, as well as being important for brain function.

Extreme signs of deficiency are muscle twitches, childhood growing pains, dizziness or a poor sense of balance, sore knees and joint pain.

The best plant sources of manganese are watercress, pineapple, endive, blackberries, raspberries, lettuce, grapes, strawberries, beetroot (beet), celery, oats, nuts and seeds.

MOLYBDENUM
Molybdenum is an essential nutrient used for detoxifying the body from free radicals and other environmental pollutants. It helps the body to get rid of the waste products from digested proteins, and it strengthens teeth.

Extreme signs of deficiency are rare in humans, although animals show signs of mental disorders and breathing difficulties.

The best plant sources are tomatoes, wholegrain products, beans and lentils.

SELENIUM

Selenium is an essential nutrient and trace mineral that impacts brain function. Glutathione is an important brain anti-oxidant, and nerve cells require selenium to produce it. A lowering of mood, including depression, and an increase in anxiety are two of the most noticeable symptoms of selenium deficiency, as well as lowered immunity. When partnered with vitamin E, its action is synergistic, which means they are more active together than when functioning alone. It is also useful for natural mercury detoxification, as it helps to break mercury down, facilitating its excretion from the body.

Extreme signs of deficiency are reduced anti-oxidant protection, cataracts, high blood pressure, frequent infections and premature ageing.

The best plant sources are mushrooms, cabbage, zucchini (courgette), avocados, lentils, seaweed and Brazil nuts.

ZINC

Zinc is a trace mineral and essential nutrient critical for cellular growth and metabolism. It is also involved in gene expression. These processes are dependant on a constant supply of zinc from the diet. During a period of rapid growth and development, which is typical in infancy and childhood, a deficiency in zinc can lead to a less than optimally developed neurological system. The role zinc plays in brain metabolism is very important as it bolsters the strength of neuronal cell membranes and helps to destroy free radicals.

Zinc also helps to get rid of lead, which can be very damaging to cognitive function. Zinc also plays a role in neurogenesis — the creation of new neurons, the maturation of neurons and the formation of synapses. It is found in large concentrations in the hippocampus, which is the seat of memory and learning in the brain. It also seems to modulate specific neurotransmitters such as glutamate and GABA receptors.

Zinc is also necessary for the conversion of alpha-linolenic and linoleic acid into essential fatty acid derivatives (eicosanoids), which are essential for brain growth, development and maintenance. Essential fatty acids are necessary for zinc to be absorbed from the gut as well. So, there is a two-way relationship between EFAs and zinc — both have to be consumed to be able to accomplish all their respective tasks.

Zinc is also required for serotonin and melatonin synthesis, which means that if it isn't supplied in the diet or if more than what the diet supplies is needed, sleep patterns and moods can be affected negatively. Anxiety is another side effect of zinc deficiency.

Extra zinc is required during specific developmental phases such as puberty and growth spurts, and when ill and experiencing stress. Men need more zinc after they reach puberty because it is concentrated in sperm.

Extreme signs of zinc deficiency include white marks on fingernails, a poor sense of taste and smell, frequent infections, stretch marks, greasy and pale skin, depression, hyperactivity and loss of appetite. Digestive challenges are also present in cases of zinc deficiency. In addition, impaired growth and development, slow wound healing, poor immunity and skin rashes such as acne and eczema are also found when zinc is deficient in the diet. Anger and hostility may also present, as well as aggressiveness and a lack of care about cleanliness and grooming.

The best plant sources of zinc are ginger root, pecan nuts, green peas, turnips, Brazil nuts, rye, oats, peanuts, almonds, pumpkin seeds (pepitas), sunflower seeds and pulses (legumes).

Recommended daily allowances versus suggested optimal nutrient allowances

Old-fashioned concepts of nutrition assess dietary needs by analyzing what is eaten and comparing it to the recommended daily allowance (RDA) for each nutrient. This method is very basic since RDAs do not exist for a number of important nutrients, don't take into account individual nutrient needs or lifestyle factors and aren't relevant in terms of what is required for optimal health.

RDAs have also been nicknamed 'ridiculous dietary arbitraries' and 'official standards of accepted levels of substandard nutrition' by researchers in this field. RDAs are set by a panel of scientists in different countries, based on what is known to prevent classic nutrient deficiency diseases, but these scientists cannot agree on a standardized recommended daily allowance for most nutrients, so this means there is often great variation between countries.

Among those who research this contentious topic, there seems to be consensus on the fact that you can get enough nutrients from a normal diet to keep you from contracting diseases such as rickets or beriberi, but most people have higher goals than that. A 2005 nutrition report titled *What We Eat in America* looked at the daily diet of nearly 9000 individuals and found that there were significant numbers of people who fell way below what the RDA suggested for a variety of vitamins and minerals. Both men and women were between 75–85 per cent below the RDA for important brain nutrients!

On the basis of this evidence, suggested optimal nutrient allowances (SONAs) have been proposed as an alternative to RDAs and are more likely to be the intake necessary to maintain optimum health. SONAs are often ten times the RDA, which is confirmed by the results of many large-scale supplement research projects. There are hundreds of scientific studies published in respected medical journals which prove that intakes of vitamins above RDA levels offer a multitude of beneficial effects — enhanced infection resistance, increased intellectual performance and a reduction in birth defects, cancer and heart disease.

Furthermore, no dietary nutrient guidelines have ever been undertaken to suggest optimal nutrient intake levels for cognitive function. We simply don't know exactly what the brain requires. We do know the brain experiences problems, visible through various symptoms, when specific nutrients fall below normal levels, but there may be other more subtle symptoms that we don't pick up.

The soil that most conventional produce is grown in is not what it used to be either. Some results of soil analysis from around the world show that American soil is depleted by about 80 per cent of its minerals and Australian soil by 60 per cent. Clearly one cannot rely on food alone to provide nutrients to sustain optimum health and wellbeing.

On average, potassium levels in fruit and vegetables have fallen by 17.5 per cent between 1940 and 2002, magnesium by 20 per cent, iron by 25.5 per cent and calcium by 31 per cent. Assessing the levels of other nutrients, such as vitamin C, shows significant declines too. On average, organic produce does result in more nutrient-dense foods, partly due to the healthier soil they are grown in which contains more nutrients the plants can absorb. A large overview of published studies and literature reviews spanning from 1980 and 2007 supports this conclusion.

One of the arguments that anti-supplement advocates use to frighten people is that high amounts of vitamins might cause an overdose. Only a few vitamins taken in excess can cause health problems and generally these would have to be taken in exclusion from other vitamins and in such excessively high dosages that it is very unlikely that anyone would do this. As an example, vitamin B6 can cause nerve damage if taken in excessive amounts. To cause this damage 1000–6000 mg per day would have to be consumed. Even a 'mega dose' B-vitamin supplement only contains 50–100 mg of this vitamin. Between 1983 and 1990, Local Poison Control Centers in the United States reported 2556 fatalities directly caused by medically prescribed drugs — but no deaths from vitamins. The latest report from the American Association of Poison Control Centers (AAPCC) attributes no deaths to vitamins in the 27 years that the report has been available.

Reasons to supplement your diet with extra vitamins and minerals

We all live in a polluted environment, from the water we drink to the air that we breathe to the chemicals that we ingest in large quantities from the foods that we eat. Our bodies are constantly trying to detoxify so that we can maintain our good health. Extra nutrients are required to keep the detoxification pathways in the body functioning well due to the ongoing exposure we have to toxins today.

The food that we eat, even if it is fresh produce, has been transported and stored before we get to eat it. Nutrient losses occur when food is harvested. If it is cooked and canned, further nutrients and enzymes are lost. Refining it, as with grains, further removes nutrients.

The food that we eat generally comes from depleted soil, which is deficient in the very nutrients that we all need in ever-increasing amounts. Remember, plant cells require most of the same nutrients that we require as humans. Because we need to grow vast quantities of food very quickly, we are left with masses of deficient food, which can fill us up and satisfy our appetite, but can't satisfy our biological requirements.

We are all experiencing inordinate amounts of stress, which bombard us from many different directions. The world we have created for ourselves is filled with situations and experiences that create feelings of anxiety, frustration and being overwhelmed. When the brain experiences stress, it requires more nutrients than a normal, good diet can fulfill.

It is much more common to have micronutrient deficiencies than excess nutrients in the body, due to the reasons above, so it makes sense to supplement wisely. There are very few cases of micronutrient overdoses, so it is safe to take out this particular form of nutritional insurance if you take the advice of a qualified nutritional practitioner.

If you are avoiding a specific group of foods due to a food intolerance or sensitivity, or because of a personal choice, then you may be missing out on a variety of good nutrients too. It is important to note that refined foods also deplete nutrients from the body in the process of digesting them simply due to the extra load they place on tissues and organs.

A vitamin and mineral supplement that meets RDA requirements may not supply the quantity required of a specific nutrient either. For example, most multivitamins contain 2–5 mg of zinc, whereas the quantity required for benefit may be closer to 15–20 mg. The same situation exists for magnesium. We all have basic requirements for vitamins and minerals but, unfortunately, environmental factors, genetic predispositions, gender and age may make us need higher amounts of particular nutrients than what a simple multivitamin provides. For example, an athlete will require more vitamins and minerals than a person who does very little exercise, and a pregnant woman will require more than a woman who is not pregnant. A simple RDA supplement may not be all you need to help your body cope with the toxins and stress that most people are exposed to today. In order to feel your best, both mentally and physically, you need a steady and consistent supply of vitamins and minerals from unprocessed foods and a good multivitamin.

If you are battling with any mood, focus, memory or sleep challenges, see a qualified naturopath or a nutrition-minded physician, either of whom can organize specific blood tests to assess your nutrient status. A practitioner will recommend the best supplement to take based on your age, gender, nutrient deficiencies, lifestyle and individual nutrient needs. Supplements are made up of synthetic versions of real nutrients, so they need to be chosen with care. See Resources on page 262.

Water and your brain

Although water isn't a nutrient, it is critically important for optimal brain function. Water is the universal solvent and carrier, which means that it has the ability to carry nutrients, such as glucose, amino acids and other nutrients, to every cell in the body and brain.

Water also flushes wastes and toxins out of cells, excreting them through the kidneys, bowel and skin. Water helps to maintain blood circulation and volume, essential functions for all tissues and organs. It also increases the capacity of haemoglobin (the red pigment in blood) to carry oxygen, which influences life at the cellular level. The digestive process requires water to break down foods, along with digestive enzymes. All these processes are necessary for optimal brain function.

However, the role that water plays directly in the brain is just as critical. Water comprises more of the brain in percentage terms than any other organ of the body, so dehydration will influence brain function. The electrical transmissions within the central nervous system enable thinking, sensory input, learning and activity. Optimal nerve and muscle function rely on membranes to have the correct polarity, which is part of the electrical transmission process. When dehydration sets in, this reduces the polarity across the membrane and in turn influences the ability of the membrane to be selective about what it responds to. When a cell has high polarity, it raises the threshold of sensitivity at the cell membrane, which increases its integrity. It becomes less sensitive to outside stimuli, which allows enhanced selective focus for learning. Research indicates that memory and attention both suffer when a brain is dehydrated and that mood is negatively affected too.

When the body and brain are dehydrated the stress hormone cortisol is released, which also stops your brain from feeling calm and in control, leading to mood swings and less than optimal cognitive function.

When you are dehydrated your body can mistake the signal for water to mean that you're hungry. Although you would imagine that the sensation of hunger and thirst are very different, and they are, eating can soothe thirst initially. In addition, dehydration leads to fatigue, which the brain can interpret as a signal to eat something that will release energy quickly, like sugar. So you end up eating something when you should be drinking water instead.

A vicious cycle is established when you confuse thirst and hunger because the more you eat, the greater your need for water becomes, as your body also needs water to manufacture digestive enzymes to break down the food you are eating. There is a simple formula to work out how much water a day you should be drinking. First, you will need to determine your weight in kilograms. If you know your weight in pounds, multiply that figure by 0.45 to convert it into kilograms. For every 10 kg of body weight you should be drinking 300 ml of water. So, for example, if you weigh 50 kg, multiply 5 x 300 to give you 1500 ml (1½ litres, roughly 3 pints, or 6 glasses).

Action plan

Five things to do that will introduce more vitamins and minerals into your diet (as well as water):

1. Make colourful salads as well as colourful pasta and stir-fried dishes. Look at your plate and make sure there are lots of greens and other colours to feed your cells.

2. Make smoothies with added fruit, nuts and seeds as well as dairy-free milks like coconut milk.

3. Eat colourful snacks that are raw and fresh, as well as fruit sticks and nut butters. Make it easy for yourself by having fresh food available at all times, as well as hummus and nut butters.

4. Wean yourself off juices and enjoy clean, fresh water.

5. Start using a natural multivitamin supplement to fill in the nutrient gaps left by deficient soil, over-stored produce and extra stress.

See the Resources section for more supportive information.

CHAPTER 5

Protein and communication in your brain

A lthough people are very seldom deficient in protein while living in developed countries, there are a number of things that can influence the digestion and absorption of protein and its effectiveness at providing the nutritional foundation for neurotransmitters, which are one of the cornerstones of the brain's communication capabilities.

A large portion of the flow of information that occurs in the central nervous system (CNS), which includes the brain, is controlled by neurotransmitters. You don't get the correct message about what is going on in your world if these tiny messengers aren't able to do their job properly.

When people think of proteins they generally think of meat, but proteins are found in many foods including plant foods. Proteins are extremely important for the processes of thinking, learning and remembering as well as stable mood maintenance. In addition, protein is also responsible for the creation of a variety of hormones, such as leptin and insulin, which are intricately involved in appetite regulation, metabolism and weight management, working both with and in the brain to accomplish these tasks.

The aim of this chapter is to give you a clear grasp of why the brain needs protein.

THE IMPORTANCE OF PROTEIN

The manufacture of hormones, such as leptin and insulin, relies on protein, and coupled with digestive enzymes, ensures stable blood glucose levels, satiation and healthy weight maintenance. Protein is also needed to make neurotransmitters, so a lack of protein will directly influence brain function.

Proteins need ... digestive enzymes to break them down into usable amino acids.

And ... protein is the foundation of hormones, one of which is insulin. So inadequte protein intake/digestion and absorption

Will lead to ... inadequte insulin and leptin production

Which leads to ... poor energy supply to cells (insulin is required to get glucose into cells for energy production), plus poor signalling to the brain that satiation has been reached (leptin tells the brain that the stomach is full).

Which leads to ... binge eating of fast-release nutrient-deficient foods in a vain attempt to get an energy boost

Which will lead to ... a further downward spiral.

It will help you understand the different types of neurotransmitters in your brain, what they do and why they need 'clean' sources of protein to function effectively.

Neurotransmitters are tiny but mighty

Neurotransmitters are tiny chemicals that relay, amplify and modulate signals between neurons. They carry information between neurons across a small space called the synaptic cleft to enable our thoughts to make sense, our emotions to be clear and our moods to be understood and reasonable. When our neurotransmitters function well, we feel good, but when they don't, a number of different challenges can arise. When you consider that neurons never actually touch their neighbours but simply communicate with an electro-chemical impulse across a tiny space, you realize how amazing the brain is.

Neurotransmitters, as part of the message they send, incorporate a signal to either 'excite' or 'inhibit' a response. However, some neurotransmitters have both excitatory and inhibitory functions, while others don't do either yet they still perform different and important tasks.

On another level, it depends on what type of neuron is sending and/or receiving the signal as to what message the neurotransmitter sends. Each neurotransmitter has a specific function and by stimulating the release of various neurotransmitters, we have a powerful mechanism to influence our thinking. For example, watching a soothing, calming scene will stimulate the release of serotonin and gamma-butyric acid (GABA), leaving you feeling serene and relaxed. Watching a frightening scene from a horror movie will stimulate the release of neurotransmitters that will leave you feeling agitated and unsettled.

The place that the neurotransmitter is absorbed into after it has crossed the synapse is called the receptor, which also determines what type of message is sent further up into the neuron. The end result is that the ultimate effect of these signalling factors is to either cause a neuron to fire or not!

Neurotransmitters perform an intricate dance

Each neurotransmitter may have many different receptors in d fferent areas of the brain. The action of these receptors will influence the action of the neurotransmitter. There are two main types of receptors: ionotrophic and metabotrophic. Ionotrophic receptors, by managing the flow of certain ions either into or out of a cell, change the polarization of the cell. This leads to either a stimulatory or inhibitory response on the receptor, which will turn a neuron's communication on or off. Metabotrophic receptors activate a specific protein which opens the ion channels directly and triggers a cascade of metabolic reactions which lead to an increase or decrease in the excitability of a neuron. Here the strength of the communication is influenced, not its activation or deactivation.

Proteins are what most neurotransmitters are made up of, so a good supply of proteins is necessary for optimal brain function. Proteins are made up of amino acids, which are the building blocks of the brain and body, along with the right kind of fats. Amino acids make specific compounds that are called precursors. These precursors get converted into neurotransmitters using specific enzymes which are dependant on vitamins and minerals.

The liver produces about 60 per cent of the amino acids we require; the other 40 per cent must be obtained from the diet. It therefore makes sense to ensure your liver stays healthy (see page 71 for more about the liver). Some amino acids are essential, meaning they have to be obtained from food, while other non-essential ones can be synthesized in the liver. However, during sickness or stress, the non-essential amino acids can become essential and need to be sourced directly from food.

Amino acids are linked together in different sequences so they can make up different brain neurotransmitters. If there is a lack of these messengers, neurons won't be able to communicate properly, leading to a variety of cognitive challenges such as depression and anxiety as well as memory, learning and concentration challenges and fluctuating levels of motivation and mental alertness.

Studies have linked low levels of certain amino acids to attention difficulties. This may be due to a number of things: an insufficient intake of protein from the diet, the inadequate transport of these essential nutrients from the digestive tract, a problem with their absorption from the digestive tract, or some problem with them being synthesized into the precursors to the neurotransmitters.

Furthermore, amino acids help to make insulin, which gets glucose out of the bloodstream into the cells. Various amino acids are also required to help cells regulate and maintain their balance of glucose. So a lack of protein will influence cellular glucose uptake and absorption, both of which will affect cognition negatively.

Protein is also required to ensure new memories are made as brain cells need protein to change their structure so memories are laid down in the hippocampus and other parts of the brain. Without enough protein, the cells required to forge memories cannot produce the required changes and memory will be impacted. Feeling bright and focused is very challenging when your brain is battling to concentrate and lay down new memories!

The top neurotransmitters

Although there are hundreds of different sequences of amino acids that make up more than 60 different neurotransmitters, here are the most important ones:

DOPAMINE, ADRENALINE AND NORADRENALINE

Dopamine, adrenaline and noradrenaline all produce a stimulating, motivating response to help with stress management and to provide a feeling of wellbeing. However, too much adrenaline can lead to excessive anxiety and exhaustion.

Dopamine is involved in the controlled movement of the body, emotional responsiveness and the ability to experience both pleasure and pain. It's often called the 'pleasure' neurotransmitter. Parkinson's disease as well as Alzheimer's disease and attention deficit disorder (ADD) have all been linked to low levels of this neurotransmitter. Dopamine is released and gives pleasure with the aim of getting you to repeat the behaviour. This is likely to be a biological adaptation as pleasure-producing experiences, such as orgasms, helped to perpetuate the species. Experiences that ended up frightening us often ended our lives, so it makes sense to repeat experiences that feel good because they are more

HOW YOUR BODY MAKES ADRENALINE

Proteins + Zinc + Vitamin B1 + Vitamin B6 + Stomach Acid

L-Phenylalanine (an amino acid)
+
Vitamin C + Iron + Vitamin B3 + Vitamin B6 + Vitamin B9 (Folate)

L-Tyrosine (an amino acid)
+
Vitamin C + Iron + Vitamin B2 + Vitamin B3 + Vitamin B9 (Folate)

L-Dopa
+
Zinc + Magnesium + Vitamin B6 + Vitamin C

Dopamine
+
Vitamin C + Copper

Noradrenaline

SAMe (S-Adenosyl Methionine) + Manganese + Phosphorous +
Vitamin B5 + Vitamin B9 (Folate)

Adrenaline

Adrenaline is a 'survival' hormone and the body uses many nutrients to synthesize it. Ongoing stress depletes you of these critical nutrients and leads to mental and physical exhaustion and faster ageing. Being calm and happy leads to more energy and a healthy brain and body.

Source: Tabrizian I. *Visual Textbook of Nutritional Medicine.* NRS Publications, Yokine, WA. 2012

likely to keep us alive! The amino acid precursor for this neurotransmitter is tyrosine and phenylalanine (the precursor of tyrosine). Vitamin B6, magnesium and zinc are all necessary for its production, although other nutrients have also been found to be important such as folic acid (vitamin B9), vitamin B3, vitamin B12 and vitamin C, as well as iron and copper.

Noradrenaline is involved in concentration, alertness, mood and the formation of memories. When it is produced in excess due to high levels of stress, it leads to feelings of extreme anxiety and even panic. It is involved in the release of hormones that stimulate the thymus gland. Precursors for this neurotransmitter are phenylalanine and tyrosine. Dopamine is the immediate precursor. Co-factors for the production of this neurotransmitter include vitamin B3 and S-adenosylmethionine (SAMe).

Adrenaline helps us respond to stress and is the fight or flight hormone, so too much of it will leave you feeling exhausted, run-down and anxious. Dopamine is the precursor to this important neurotransmitter.

Symptoms of deficiency in these neurotransmitters include caffeine and/or sugar cravings, light-headedness or dizziness, fatigue, reduced libido, pale skin, depression, being overweight, and movement disorders such as Parkinson's disease.

Food sources for the precursors to these important neurotransmitters are high protein foods like beef, pork, fish and tofu. Other sources include pumpkin seeds (pepitas), avocado, black-eyed and pinto beans.

GABA (GAMMA-AMINOBUTYRIC ACID)

GABA counteracts the stimulating neurotransmitters dopamine, adrenaline and noradrenaline leading to feelings of relaxation and calmness, especially after stress. Lack of GABA has been implicated in disturbed sleep, as well as drug and alcohol addiction. Should you be deficient in vitamin B6 and have high levels of glutamine, the conversion process will stop at glutamate and it will not convert to GABA. Glutamate is an excitatory neurotransmitter, so you will be left feeling anxious and unsettled. Alcohol and anxiolytic drugs boost GABA's effects, which is why they are very addictive.

Symptoms of GABA deficiency include twitching, trembling, restlessness, carbohydrate cravings, heart palpitations, sweating, clammy and/or cold hands, a lump in the throat, anxiety, butterflies in the stomach, digestive challenges, tinnitus and premenstrual syndrome (PMS).

Food sources for the precursor to this important neurotransmitter are wholegrains, nuts, lentils, citrus fruit, broccoli, banana and spinach.

SEROTONIN

Serotonin works to regulate sleep, mood and eating behaviours. It also helps you feel safe and secure. Vitamin B3, vitamin B6, vitamin C as well as magnesium and zinc are important for its production from tryptophan. If you are deficient in B vitamins, your body's ability to produce serotonin will be severely compromised. Serotonin stimulates the release of endogenous opioids (endorphins), which are compounds that allow us to feel blissful and euphoric. When we exercise endorphins are released, which is why we feel so good after a strenuous workout. Most antidepressants artificially boost this neurotransmitter.

Symptoms of serotonin deficiency include headache, backache, sleep disorders, depression, anorexia, bulimia, hyper vigilance, shortness of breath and salt cravings.

Food sources for the precursors (tryptophan) to this important neurotransmitter are turkey, sunflower seeds, salmon, potato, Swiss cheese, cottage cheese, brown rice, banana and mackerel; however, tryptophan is only found in very small quantities in these foods. As a consequence, it doesn't always cross the blood–brain barrier in the quantities required for optimal benefit. This is why a supplement may be required if you are experiencing deficiency symptoms.

ACETYLCHOLINE

Acetylcholine has a stimulating action and assists in memory function, concentration, learning ability and cognitive alertness. It's also involved in sleep and the movement of muscles, so whenever you move, this neurotransmitter is being released. Choline is the precursor for this neurotransmitter, with co-factors for its production including vitamins B1 and B5, vitamin C as well as magnesium. The compound acetyl-L-carnitine can also facilitate synthesis.

Symptoms of deficiency include difficulty concentrating and paying attention, memory challenges, fat cravings, a dry mouth and cough.

Food sources for the precursors to this important neurotransmitter are cabbage, cauliflower, almonds, blueberries, cheese, chicken, eggs, broad beans (fava beans), peanut butter and grape juice.

MELATONIN

Melatonin keeps the body and mind in sync with whether it's day or night, and is produced from serotonin. If you don't have enough serotonin, you won't get enough melatonin being produced. Interestingly, it also acts as an anti-oxidant, which is one of the reasons why sleep is so important for optimal health. Serotonin is also produced in greater quantities during the summer months due to the action of the sun on the pineal gland, which increases its production. This is thought to be part of the explanation for seasonal affective disorder (SAD), where some people experience mood disturbances, such as apathy and depression, in the months when there is less sunlight.

Symptoms of melatonin deficiency include sleep challenges as well as mood challenges such as sadness and depression.

Food sources for the precursors to this important neurotransmitter are not vast, with cherries being first in line and then red grapes. As the body can make melatonin from serotonin, it may be best to focus on food sources for serotonin rather than searching for cherries, which are out of season most of the year. Cherry juice, if not sweetened, may be a good alternative.

Neurotransmitters are like Goldilocks because ...

As you can see from the list above, neurotransmitters balance each other out. There has to be a very fine balance between the excitatory and inhibitory neurotransmitters, because if only one type is active, we'll either be excessively excited and distracted or unable to move or accomplish anything. One must produce a stimulating response, while another must produce a calming response and they need to be able to do this harmoniously otherwise the brain will be haphazard and confusion will reign.

When protein is eaten and absorbed well, the digestive process will break down the protein into amino acids and they will become messengers, telling the neurons what to do at the appropriate time. For example, when you are reading a book and need to concentrate, the messages sent to the appropriate neurons will help your brain to lock out interfering noises and focus on the words on the page. If the messages are not getting to where they need to go, the focus and concentration required to block out the noises in the environment will not be available.

The balance and maintenance of these neurotransmitters is an important part of mental wellbeing.

For neurotransmitters to work properly, the precursors (the amino acids) have to be supplied by the diet in levels that accumulate in the blood plasma. The amount of each precursor that reaches the brain via the blood–brain barrier is dependent on the levels in the blood plasma. This is why it is important to get an adequate intake of protein from food.

In addition, if the liver is not operating optimally, amino-acid production will be compromised, leading to reduced neurotransmitter function.

Once the precursor is in the brain, various enzymes will convert it into the neurotransmitter it's meant to be. The enzyme will then be set free to repeat the process again when required. The final step in the life of a neurotransmitter is to be broken down and removed from the synaptic cleft after its job has been performed. This is an important part in the whole process, otherwise it would continue to 'excite' or 'inhibit' actions over and over again. This beautiful and intricate dance occurs over and over again, and when working optimally has the potential to lead to stable mood, clear thought and emotional balance — a natural lightness and brightness!

feed
your
brain

HOW THE BODY MAKES YOU HAPPY
(AND THEN SLEEPY)

Proteins
+
Zinc + Vitamin B1 + Vitamin B6 + Stomach Acid

L-Tryptophan (an amino acid – a small protein)
+
Iron + Calcium + Vitamin B3 + Vitamin B9 (Folate)

5-Hydroxytryptophan (5-HTP)
+
Vitamin B6 + Vitamin C + Magnesium + Zinc

5-Hydroxytryptamine (Serotonin)

TO MAKE MELATONIN FROM SEROTONIN
+
Proteins + Zinc + Vitamin B1 + Vitamin B6 + Stomach Acid

Methionine
+
Magnesium

SAMe (S-adenosylmethionine)
+
Vitamin B5

Melatonin

Serotonin is a very important neurotransmitter that makes you feel happy and secure. To be able to fall asleep with ease at night, your body needs the nutrients required to make serotonin, so that it can be converted into melatonin when darkness falls.

Source: Tabrizian I. *Visual Textbook of Nutritional Medicine*. NRS Publications, Yokine, WA, 2012.

Parkinson's disease

A clear example of a loss of neurotransmitter function (or rather dysfunction) is in the development of Parkinson's disease. In this progressive illness, the amount of dopamine is reduced in the brain leading to cognitive dysfunction and the individual being unable to control their movements. This is the result of not just the dopamine system working incorrectly but also other systems, such as the GABA and acetylcholine systems, which all work together to initiate and inhibit movement. Researchers believe that the imbalance that occurs between various neurotransmitters is one of the causes of cognitive dysfunction in ageing people. The lack of smooth, uninterrupted neurotransmitter function leads to various complications including Parkinson's disease.

What about protein powders?

Protein shakes, bars and powders may not be the miracle products they seem to be. When protein is 'isolated' in protein powders and energy bars, the amino acids are no longer in the form that nature intended us to use them. This is what the term 'isolated' means.

Two different processes are used to produce isolated protein powders: acid hydrolysis and fermentation. Both of these processes produce impurities that some people react negatively to, especially if they are also sensitive to MSG.

When you read the labels of these products you will notice that the quantity of the amino acids glutamate and aspartate are very high. This is problematic for the brain because the brain dislikes these two amino acids in such a concentrated form.

You may recall that MSG (monosodium glutamate) is a toxic additive that should be avoided. The isolated glutamate in protein powders and bars is bad for the same reason: glutamate is a neurotransmitter that excites the brain cells. When it is supplied to the brain in normal quantities, such as in unprocessed, natural and fresh foods, then it is quite harmless because it is mildly stimulating and the brain uses it naturally. However, in its isolated form, such as in protein powders, glutamate may be dangerous to the brain because it overstimulates the excitatory action of the neurotransmitter causing cell death in the long term. Aspartate, which is also found in certain sugar replacements and is similar to aspartame in action, poses the same threat to the brain.

It is therefore best to obtain protein from real foods or from supplements that contain an unprocessed form of protein, such as hemp protein. These proteins are recognized by the body as real food and support optimal brain health.

Neurotransmitters don't work alone

The messages that move between neurons and around the brain cannot do their job properly if the brain is lacking in the right fats because the right fats help the messages jump between neurons. The brain also needs the right kind of carbohydrates to keep the neurons energized otherwise they won't have the energy to carry the messages.

The ability of neurotransmitters to communicate properly is dependant on the amount of fatty acids in the membrane. Changes in these fatty acids can affect the function of the receptors and enzymes that are responsible for the neurotransmission that occurs between neurons.

Vitamins and minerals are also important for the correct synthesis of neurotransmitters, as they act as co-factors in the production of these important communicators. If there are inadequate amounts of various vitamins or minerals, the production of neurotransmitters will be negatively influenced. Vitamins and minerals help to make the enzymes needed to keep the messages strong and focused. They also help the fats to work optimally and the carbohydrates to energize the brain. This can only be achieved if digestion and the absorption of nutrients are performing ideally (see page 48).

Folic acid is a very important nutrient

Folic acid, also known as vitamin B9, is an extremely important nutrient for optimal brain function (see page 86), however it needs to be changed via specific enzymes to be able to perform its tasks properly. A specific gene called MTHFR produces an enzyme called methylenetetrahydrofolate reductase, which converts folic acid into methylfolate. This compound is extremely important for optimal brain function because it is involved in the synthesis of neurotransmitters and s-adenosylmethionine (SAMe). SAMe regulates more than 200 different enzymes in the body and is involved in neurotransmitter production. A lack of SAMe is linked to serious health challenges such as cancer, Down syndrome and autism. Many people have a MTHFR gene that doesn't work properly. This means that it will produce a less effective enzyme, resulting in less effective folic acid conversion. The end result is a lowered capacity for optimal neurotransmitter synthesis. Poor lifestyle choices, as well as a toxic environment are thought to be involved in the changes on the MTHFR gene. Screening for this polymorphism is available (see Resources on page 262).

What about antidepressants?

There are a number of different antidepressants available today and each one differs in the way it affects the balance and function of specific neurotransmitters. Although there are differences in their mechanisms of action, antidepressants have some things in common: they are effective in 50–80 per cent of users (although some recent studies are suggesting these figures may be inflated and they may be particularly dangerous when used in adolescence), they take from six to eight weeks to produce full effects, and their side effects can be severe.

Tricyclic antidepressants (TCAs) are one of the oldest types of these medications. They prevent the re-uptake of serotonin and noradrenaline, which extends the presence of these chemicals in the synapse, prolonging the mood-lightening effect of these drugs. A newer type of antidepressant called SSRIs (selective serotonin re-uptake inhibitors) blocks the re-uptake of serotonin so that there is more of it available, which leads to mood elevation. Some research indicates an increased risk of bone fracture in adults over the age of 50 who use this form of antidepressant.

Monoamine oxidase inhibitors (MAOIs) reduce the level of the enzyme monoamine oxidase in the synapse. This enzyme normally breaks down serotonin and noradrenaline, so lower levels of the enzyme leads to higher amounts of serotonin and noradrenaline in the body. RIMAs (reversible inhibitors of monoamine oxidase type A) have a similar action, but only work with one of the inhibitors and have fewer dietary restrictions.

Noradrenaline re-uptake inhibitors (NARIs) elevate the level of the neurotransmitter norepinephrine in the synapse by inhibiting its re-uptake. In so doing, it makes more of this neurotransmitter available, which helps the user to feel better. NaSSAs or SNRIs (noradrenergic and specific serotonergic antidepressants) are one of the newest types of antidepressants and work on both serotonin and noradrenaline by blocking their receptors to prolong the mood-lifting effect of released serotonin and noradrenaline.

Unfortunately, all of these medications are not without side effects, which include a dry mouth, weight gain, constipation, headaches, sleep difficulties, skin rashes, blurred vision, hand tremors and anxiety. There are researchers who believe that simply increasing the neurotransmitters naturally through specific supplements is a better way to treat mood disorders rather than stopping the re-uptake of these neurotransmitters. Others believe it is the neuron's actual axon and dendrite (from which the neurotransmitters are released) that are damaged and that supplemented essential fatty acids may help alleviate depression. This theory is well supported by research.

How drugs work in your brain

You now understand that some neurotransmitters are able to excite certain neuronal responses while others inhibit them. Some clever ones can do both on different occasions. The receptor on the neuron's axon is what a neurotransmitter attaches to when it finds the right lock to fit into. The receptor is the most important place to a psychoactive drug because a receptor doesn't know whether a drug or a neurotransmitter is fitting into its lock. All it knows is whether the key is the right one and many drugs imitate neurotransmitters to fool the receptor into responding and becoming activated. These kinds of drugs are called agonists (such as heroin and nicotine) and bind to the opioid receptors that control pain and pleasure and magnify feelings of wellbeing and euphoria. Antagonist drugs, on the other hand, block the activity of specific neurotransmitters (such as naloxone which is used to counter the effects of heroin overdose).

Neurotransmitters and mood-altering drugs

Mood-altering substances, which stimulate the production of specific neurotransmitters, lead to the brain becoming reliant on them. This occurs because these substances result in your brain shutting down its own production of these specific neurotransmitters in its aim to maintain balance at all times. If too many substances are supplied from an unnatural

114

source, such as a drug, then the brain compensates for this excess by stopping its own natural production of this neurotransmitter. Unfortunately, when this occurs on an ongoing basis, the brain ends up being reliant on an external, unnatural supply of the substance, which in turn relies on more and more of the substance to get the same sensation or feeling.

This is why addiction is so insidious and dangerous and why getting off a mood-altering substance is very difficult. Researchers in this field believe that if you don't correct the chemical balance in the brain after the person is free of their addiction, they have a much greater chance of succumbing to the addictive substance again.

Eat a variety of proteins

When you choose a wide variety of proteins from different sources, your brain is capable of making all the necessary neurotransmitters for optimal cognitive function. Animal products contain protein as do legumes, nuts and seeds. Combining lentils and rice, for example, produces an improved quality of protein in the form of a full complement of amino acids, because lentils are high in the amino acids that rice is low in.

Animal forms of protein are fine in small quantities, but they lack fibre and can be quite constipating if consumed in excess. Adding more plant protein to your diet adds fibre as well as some nutrients that animal products are low in, such as phytonutrients.

Plant forms of protein are also more colourful. There is a lot of research to indicate that vegetarians can be just as healthy as their meat-eating peers, if enough care is taken to include a variety of proteins, grains, nuts and seeds in their diet. If you are pursuing a vegan or vegetarian diet, you must watch for any iron and vitamin B12 deficiency as they are common in these cases. Plant forms of iron are not as easily assimilated as animal forms of iron (see page 90), and vitamin B12 is not found in plants (see page 80).

Vegetarians can make sure they get enough protein by including seed foods in their diet. These are foods that would grow if they were planted, including nuts, seeds, legumes, quinoa and maize (corn). Broccoli and cauliflower are also 'seed' foods, so they should form part of your regular diet as well.

When selecting protein foods, organic products are best because they are 'cleaner' than conventional protein products, containing fewer toxins and pesticides as well as no antibiotics or hormones if it is an animal form of protein. These compounds place a toxic load on your brain. Conventionally grown meat contains about fourteen times more pesticides than plant foods, and dairy products have five-and-a-half times more. Animal-origin foods have greatly concentrated amounts of chemicals in them, simply because they are at the top of the food chain. When you choose to prepare and serve more plant-based foods, you are naturally less exposed to chemical contamination. Your ability to feel light and bright is increased substantially when your toxic load is reduced.

Choose animal products with care

Animal products require careful preservation to stay fresh and to prevent serious contamination and illness. However, some of the preservatives used to keep meat fresh are questionable in terms of their long-term health effects. Here are a few pointers to keep in mind when purchasing animal flesh.

Ground or mince meat can be a mixture of various different types of meat from different carcasses. It may also be a combination of flesh from the inside and outside of the animal, posing serious contamination risks. It is best to buy your own meat and 'process' it yourself.

Processed meats, such as bacon, salami, sausages and cold cuts are conveniently prepared, sliced and preserved. They are not fresh and contain a number of troublesome additives like preservatives, dyes, excess salt and even sugar. A special type of preservative called sodium nitrite has been used in preserved meats for many years. When foods that contain nitrites are heated, these compounds change into nitrosamines, which have been linked to various forms of cancer including brain tumours, as well as insulin resistance. Nitrites also convert into nitrosamines in the digestive tract in the absence of antioxidants. Nitrates found naturally in fresh produce, such as vegetables, convert into small quantities of nitrites in the body. Researchers believe that the added vitamins and minerals that come in fresh produce stop them from being dangerous to our health. Sodium nitrate (known as Chile saltpeter or Peru saltpeter) is also used in fertilizers as well as a preservative and colour enhancer in processed meats.

Processed meats contain on average four times as much salt as unprocessed meat and up to 50 per cent more nitrites. Even processed meat that is labelled 'natural' may contain hidden nitrites. Furthermore, research has shown that mothers who ate cured meats containing nitrosamines (especially hot dogs and sausages) during pregnancy increased the risk of their children getting brain tumours. Interestingly, this was known nearly 50 years ago when researchers showed that more than 100 nitrosamines are carcinogenic and no animal species, including the monkey, proved to be resistant to nitrosamine carcinogenesis.

Grain-fed beef is the kind of meat that the majority of people eat today, simply because grains are much cheaper to feed to animals and very few animals have access to their natural food in feedlots. Grains provide the animal with food that enables quick growth and fat accumulation, and then provides the consumer with the fats present in the grains, mostly omega-6s. Choose grass-fed meat instead.

Chicken isn't what it used to be either. A study in 2004 found that chicken contained twice as much fat as it did in 1940, which means that it doesn't contain as much protein as most people assume it does. Chicken nuggets are obviously even worse with the chicken off-cuts being used as well as fillers and damaging fats. So eating free-range, organic chicken is the best choice.

Eggs are a good source of protein, but you should make an effort to purchase organic and free-range eggs. These will be free of hormones and antibiotics, both of which your brain can do without.

Goat's cheese is a good source of protein, calcium and is more easily digested than dairy or cow's cheese. It also has the advantage of not containing any colours, if it is a pure cheese. Organic goat's cheese is the better choice.

Signs of protein deficiency

General poor health along with a lack of energy, digestive and sleep challenges, problems with skin, nails and hair, emotional and nervous distress as well as metabolic disorders are signs of either a lack of protein or a disturbance in its digestion and/or absorption. Distinct memory challenges are also a sign of protein deficiency, so it may be necessary to have your amino-acid profile checked by a qualified nutritional practitioner.

Research has linked early malnutrition, which includes a lack of protein, to both behavioural difficulties and lowered cognitive ability. Remember that digestive difficulties can impair the digestion of protein. This means that even though you may be eating enough protein, you are not digesting or absorbing it and therefore not making enough of the amino acids required for cell function. This lack of amino acids will lead to lowered neurotransmitter levels and neuronal communication will be hampered. Digestive enzymes can help with protein breakdown, although a more thorough digestive health approach may be required. (See page 49 for more information about digestive health.)

Action plan

Five things to do that will introduce more 'clean' protein and plant protein to your diet are:

1. Replace cold cuts with real meat and choose organic meat. This will ensure the animal products you eat are free from nitrates, nitrites and other additives such as pesticides, hormones and antibiotics.

2. Ensure you start your day with a well-balanced breakfast that includes a portion size of protein, and ensure you are getting enough protein with each snack and meal that you consume throughout the day.

3. Add legumes such as beans, lentils or chickpeas (garbanzo beans) to two of your meals, starting this week. Initially eat small quantities to get used to the new taste and to increase your exposure to plant forms of protein. Add nuts and seeds to salads or eat pesto to get more plant protein.

4. Cook the usual dishes you already enjoy such as spaghetti bolognese, but add a few red kidney beans or other legumes to get these new foods into your diet.

5. Add a pure, unprocessed form of protein, such as hemp protein, to smoothies, enjoy a nut butter with fresh fruit, or eat nuts and seeds as snacks.

See the Resources section for more supportive information.

CHAPTER 6

Stable energy for your brain

There is very little space in the brain to store energy. If you want your brain to work effectively, you will have to learn to eat well so that it doesn't run out of energy and 'forget' to store important information. When you eat for brain energy, you keep your brain working efficiently, your moods remain stable and you increase your learning and memory capacity.

It is wonderful to observe someone changing their choice of carbohydrates and feeling the difference it makes to their energy levels, their mood and their ability to focus and concentrate. Very few people know that the brain is the most energy-hungry organ in the human body, using up to half of the carbohydrates we eat to supply its voracious appetite. Learning to respect and work with its need for energy can transform your brain's ability to support you optimally.

The aim of this chapter is to explain the role carbohydrates play in energizing the brain and why you should be eating specific carbohydrates and avoiding others. It also outlines the differences between various types of sugars and how they affect the brain.

What is sugar?

When we discuss sugar we are actually discussing carbohydrates, which can be classified into two groups: simple or complex carbohydrates. Simple carbohydrates are those that are easy to digest and quickly become glucose in your bloodstream. They are the kind that we do not need a lot of and should only be eaten occasionally. The normal white sugar that people use in coffee and tea, to bake and cook with and consume in vast quantities in processed foods is a simple carbohydrate. It comes from refining either sugar cane, sugar beets or corn. The process produces various forms of sugar including molasses, dark brown sugar, raw sugar and white sugar, all of which are basically sucrose.

The second kind, complex carbohydrates, should be eaten regularly. Complex carbohydrates convert to glucose slowly in the body and are good for the brain because they supply a slow and steady stream of energy. There are no sugar highs that lead to a sugar low. Complex carbohydrates, such as grains, legumes and vegetables, as well as most fruits are what the brain thrives on.

What's the difference between glucose, fructose and sucrose?

Although there are many types of sugar, they all have some important differences. Glucose is the type of sugar the body uses for energy. It is a single sugar molecule or a monosaccharide. Fructose is also a monosaccharide, but when naturally extracted from fruit, is not good for the body. Corn also contains fructose. Sucrose is made up of two sugar molecules joined together — a glucose and a fructose molecule — which is called a disaccharide. Sugar cane and sugar beets contain sucrose. When consumed, sucrose gets converted into glucose and fructose in the body. The body can use the glucose, but stores the fructose as fat.

In addition, carbohydrates are molecules that contain both hydrogen and carbon in specific patterns, as well as starches. Starches are made up of thousands of glucose molecules joined together and the body is well suited to eating them if they are not refined.

The brain's need for glucose via carbohydrates

The brain's preferred food or fuel is glucose, which is what carbohydrates and starch get converted into. We know that carbohydrates and starches provide energy, but eaten in excess will lead to weight gain because excess carbohydrates get converted into fat. This in turn will affect brain function. Eating non-starchy carbohydrates and lots of green vegetables will provide the healthy carbohydrates the brain needs with none of the disadvantages that come from starch and refined carbohydrates. Therefore, the kind of carbohydrates you choose to eat is critically important.

Low-carbohydrate diets

A process in the liver called gluconeogenesis produces carbohydrates from specific amino acids (proteins) when we don't eat enough carbohydrates. It is an important mechanism because it ensures continued brain function by maintaining stable blood glucose levels in extreme conditions such as fasting, starvation, extreme exercise and eating a low-carbohydrate diet. Obviously, fasting or starvation will not provide long-term health and will eventually lead to death. Whether a low-carbohydrate diet is a suitable long-term approach to optimal mental health has still not been established, as there are no longitudinal research studies to refer to.

What do brain cells do with glucose?

The mitochondria are tiny energy factories in all our cells. They work very hard in the brain creating energy from oxygen and glucose. The energy 'currency' they produce is called ATP (adenosine triphosphate). As the brain can't store much energy, its cells therefore rely on a constant, steady supply of ATP for optimal functioning. The smooth flowing, cell-to-cell signalling that occurs at faster-than-light speeds between your neurons is enhanced when these mitochondria are supplied with all the nutrients they need. When they are deprived of energy, they find it difficult to build memory traces, learn new tasks, concentrate effectively and help maintain an even mood. They run out of energy when you experience blood sugar dips.

As noted previously, glucose is a simple sugar that circulates around the body via the bloodstream. If there is a lack of glucose in the bloodstream, brain function will be affected. Symptoms associated with this are tiredness, depression, aggression, irritability, forgetfulness, difficulty concentrating and emotional outbursts.

Although the brain uses glucose for energy, too much at once can be problematic. The pancreas secretes insulin, which helps glucose enter the cells to provide energy. During each meal the pancreas knows how much insulin to release even before digestion and absorption have occurred. Refined carbohydrates will cause the pancreas to produce a lot of insulin very quickly, shunting it into the cells and liver (for storage) to protect the brain from glucose or sugar overload. Eventually the pancreas gets tired of doing this, meal after meal, day in and day out, and Type 2 diabetes is the result. Having this disease increases your chances of getting dementia by 50 per cent!

The type of sugar or carbohydrate consumed will influence how quickly blood sugar levels drop and to what extent. Processed foods, including sugar (a simple carbohydrate), do not have to be converted into glucose and have very little fibre to slow down the process of absorption, thereby causing the bloodstream to be suddenly overloaded with glucose. After this quick rise in blood sugar, the blood sugar level will fall quickly and dramatically with an accompanying energy slump called reactive hypoglycaemia. This is why concentrated forms of sugar (such as lollies/candy and soda drinks) are not ideal sources of glucose for your brain because they give a big spurt of energy followed by a big drop a short while later.

Complex carbohydrates do the opposite and are the best choice for even blood glucose levels and therefore optimal brain function.

Coconut oil and brain health

The role of coconut oil in improving brain health has made many people excited about its potential to reverse brain ageing. Ketones are a type of high-energy fuel that is produced in the liver and which the brain can use as energy if there is not enough glucose available. If the brain is not capable of using glucose efficiently, due to insulin insensitivity within neurons, then the brain can be starved of energy. The medium-chain fatty acids that coconuts contain are converted into ketones by the liver and can be used by the brain when glucose levels run low, or when ageing results in impaired neuronal insulin function within the brain. Ketones have been found to be useful as an anti-epileptic nutritional strategy, along with a low-carbohydrate diet. However, there are no long-term research studies to show they can solve severe memory challenges, although there have been some promising case studies.

Blood glucose and stress

Unfortunately, the stress response can also impact your blood glucose levels. When blood glucose levels drop too low, the adrenals glands are stimulated to produce cortisol, which stimulates glucose release from the liver to keep the brain fuelled. This leads to irritability, lethargy or hyperactivity, a lack of focus and general mood disturbances. Ongoing stress keeps this cycle going, leading to an increased desire for refined carbohydrates with their quick release of energy but poor staying power.

Eating highly processed foods leads to raised insulin levels, which in turn stimulates your nervous system, leading to feelings of anxiety and stress.

Furthermore, being hungry will also lead to adrenaline release because hunger is perceived as stress for the body. This response will produce an energy surge as the body naturally accesses glucose stores in an attempt to gain energy, but it will not last and you will feel drained shortly after. Therefore, keeping healthy snacks at hand for yourself helps to keep your brain nourished and calm naturally. Of course, stable blood glucose levels from well-chosen carbohydrates at main meals (with the right fats) will ensure stable moods on an ongoing basis, and may obviate the need for snacks entirely.

Two types of blood glucose challenges

There are two kinds of blood glucose dysfunctions that can occur, with each influencing the brain in different ways.

The first is hypoglycaemia, which is alarming and life-threatening if it occurs regularly and for a sustained period. This is caused by a lack of glucose in the brain and body. The symptoms experienced with this type of blood glucose challenge are shakiness, dizziness, muscle weakness and fatigue. The production of glucagon, epinephrine, growth hormone and cortisol are increased when you experience hypoglycaemia. Should this condition be prolonged, permanent damage to the brain can occur, with neuronal function and therefore behaviour being affected.

Hyperglycaemia is the second type of blood glucose dysfunction and refers to a condition where too much blood glucose is circulating in the blood and brain. This is what is caused by Type 2 diabetes because the cells have become unresponsive to insulin and this prevents the body from converting glucose into glycogen (a stored form of glucose), which makes it difficult for the body to remove excess blood sugar from the bloodstream. The body needs to keep glucose levels at particular levels for optimum performance, and when this balance goes wrong, hyperglycaemia results.

How insulin affects your brain

Hyperinsulinemia is the technical name for reduced insulin sensitivity. This condition can be present for many years before full-blown diabetes is diagnosed. When this condition is present, there is a reduction of insulin passing across the blood–brain barrier, which means that insulin is not present in the brain in the quantities that is required to get glucose into the neurons.

Hyperglycaemia is more damaging than hypoglycaemia because too much glucose circulating in the bloodstream damages the blood vessels as well as the organs they supply blood to. This is where damage to the brain comes in because the normal functioning and survival of neurons is negatively influenced by excess circulating glucose. In addition, insulin has a protective role to play in terms of neuronal health because it influences a neuron's ability to withstand toxic insults and its ability to regenerate.

Refined sugar can be addictive

Animal studies show that a diet high in refined sugars causes changes in the reward and pleasure centres of the brain, similar to those changes caused by drugs of addiction such as heroin, cocaine and morphine. When animals are fed sucrose, they are most likely to self-administer these drugs again. Similar research indicates that sugar may be much more addictive than cocaine.

In humans a similar situation occurs, and as children we learn very quickly that the feelings that sugar produces are pleasant and we want to feel them again. Researchers believe that the mere taste of sugar leads to opiate release via our taste buds, which sends impulses through the nerves leading to the base of the brain that stimulate the brain's pleasure system leading to an association between sugar and pleasant feelings. Unfortunately, this also leads to a learned response, whereby emotions can be manipulated by reaching for another sugary treat.

Some people may be more sensitive to sugar than others, which would present as having a serious sweet tooth and the desire to eat sweet foods many times every day. Removing sugar from your diet can therefore result in the classic cravings that accompany illicit drug withdrawal, which is why the process of removing sugar should be slow and consistent, as mentioned in the action plan at the end of this chapter.

An interesting relationship between sugar and fat ...

A fascinating experiment using rats resulted in an unexpected finding: the right fats can help a brain that's high on sugar! Two groups of rats were tested to see how well they navigated a maze. One group of rats was fed a sugary diet for six weeks, while the other was fed healthy food. After six weeks, the two groups were tested on how well they could recall the maze route. The rats fed a sugary diet were slower than they'd been before, indicating their neurons were battling to talk to each other, thus disrupting the rats' ability to recall the route they'd learnt six weeks prior to their sugary diet.

Feeding rats a diet deficient in omega-3 fatty acids prior to a sugary diet also led to memory deficits in a similar experiment, while consuming omega-3s with a sugary diet enhanced their memory recall. Although these experiments were conducted on rats, it may be that humans will have the same results, as we have similar brain chemistry to rats.

What's all the fuss about breakfast?

For good brain health you need to eat breakfast. Your brain has been deprived of food for a whole night, which is usually a good ten to twelve hours if your last meal was at 7 p.m. In the morning, your brain is in need of nutrients and fuel to be able to navigate the day. A brain that is starved of fuel will make poor nutritional choices later in the day, probably by mid-morning. It is much easier to eat the double chocolate chip muffin when your brain is desperate for food than if you have eaten breakfast and now have a raw snack on hand.

And if your day has to start with coffee or tea instead of breakfast, you may need to think about what this is doing to your brain. Any beverage that artificially produces a sense of energy, like the caffeine in coffee and tea does, is not going to be helping your brain in the long term. After all, your body produces the feeling of energy using resources that are already depleted, which will then leave you feeling even more tired later on in the day, ensuring that you will reach for another cup of 'energy'. Your brain deserves nutrients to optimize its functioning, not a quick energy 'high' that quickly drops off again. In addition, caffeine can lead to anxiety, which can stimulate emotional eating, which is generally directed towards highly refined, sugary 'treats' which do not support optimal brain function.

Consuming a good breakfast of the right fats combined with unrefined carbohydrates and clean protein will lead to stable blood glucose levels and positive cognitive benefits. The right type of breakfast will be discussed in the next chapter.

The six worst artificial sweeteners

All artificial sweeteners are additives. They are produced with the primary aim of providing a sensation of sweetness in the mouth without the calories that refined sugar provides. The sweet taste primes your brain to expect something satisfying and when nothing arrives it pushes you to consume more. In addition, it increases your sweet tooth by making it much harder to avoid very sweet foods. In fact, artificial sweeteners can increase the desire for sweet foods. There is also no long-term, impartial research to show that they are safe for human consumption, and they may be very powerful neurotoxins too. Aspartame may be especially dangerous because it becomes an excitotoxin when ingested, the activity of which

COFFEE

Contains caffeine

Gets converted into

Dopamine (feel-good/pleasure neurotransmitter)
BUT
Blocks adenosine (natural brain sedative)
AND
Dopamine gets converted into

Adrenaline
BUT
Adrenaline causes

Quick rise in blood sugar

Blood sugar ups and downs
AND

DESIRE FOR MORE FEEL-GOOD CAFFEINE STIMULATION

HOW COFFEE WORKS

Coffee provides a quick dopamine pleasure-hit, but then becomes a strong stimulant when it gets converted into adrenaline. Unfortunately, this quick energy-fix is also addictive, so many people end up relying on it for energy.

leads to neuronal death over time (see page 64 for more details).

The following artificial sweeteners should be avoided if you care about optimal brain health and function: acesulfame-K (950) which is 200 times sweeter than sugar; aspartame (951) which is 200 times sweeter than sugar; cyclamate (952) which is 30 to 50 times sweeter than sugar; neotame (961) which is 7000 to 13,000 times sweeter than sugar; saccharin (954) which is 200 to 700 times sweeter than sugar; and sucralose (955) which is 600 times sweeter than sugar.

In addition, research has found that some artificial sweeteners lower the levels of serotonin in the brain of rats. Researchers believe this may also occur in the human brain. Remember, serotonin is the neurotransmitter that not only makes us feel safe and secure, but also converts into melatonin to make us sleepy and helps to regulate appetite.

Excitotoxins

An excitotoxin is a specific type of amino acid (protein) that can when it comes into contact with neurons, cause them to fire repeatedly and maintain this 'excited' state. It can cause the death of sensitive neurons. Excitotoxins are found naturally in certain foods and also in some processed foods. Artificial sweeteners as well as monosodium glutamate (MSG) are two types of excitotoxins prevalent in foods today. Researchers have found that the neurons that are particularly susceptible to Alzheimer's disease are also the neurons that use glutamate and aspartate as their neurotransmitters — two excitotoxins, which indicates that excitotoxin damage could be linked to Alzheimer's disease.

The many names for sugar

It would be simple to avoid added sugar in foods if there weren't so many different names for it. Here are a few of the names used in food products to describe 'sugar': raw sugar, molasses, cane-juice crystals, corn sweeteners, high fructose corn syrup (HFCS), honey, malted grain syrup, maple syrup, agave syrup, date sugar, coconut palm sugar, buttered syrup, caramel, carob syrup, dextran, dextrose, diastase, diastatic malt, ethyl maltol, maltitol, glucose, golden syrup, invert syrup, lactose, maltodextrin, maltose, mannitol, refiner's syrup or golden syrup, sorbitol, sorghum syrup and sucrose. The most processed sugars are the ones you should avoid, while consuming natural forms of sugar is fine in moderation.

High fructose corn syrup

A truly evil processed sugar is high fructose corn syrup (HFCS), which is a man-made, mostly glucose/dextrose substance with half of its sweetness coming in the form of fructose. It is much cheaper to manufacture than sugar, so it has naturally replaced many sugars in food. It also allows suppliers to super-size their meals at the same cost of a normal size. It is therefore not surprising that the use of this sweetener is rising in soda drinks, fruit juices and bakery items. There are two things about this sweetener that you should keep in mind: it does not stimulate the appetite-regulating hormone leptin, which tells your brain that you are getting full; and in liquid form in a sugar-laced drink it is not registered by the body in the same way that sugar in a solid form is. Therefore, weight gain and soda drink consumption have the finger pointing directly at HFCS.

Natural sweeteners

Using natural sweeteners means avoiding the brain health pitfalls of processed sugar. The best natural sweeteners have four things in common:

1. They contain vitamins and minerals, which are necessary for their metabolism.

2. They are produced using simple, chemical-free processing techniques.

3. They are derived from a natural source that should be organically grown.

4. They contain maltose and complex carbohydrates that break down more slowly in the body than the simple sugars sucrose, glucose and fructose.

If you must eat sweet foods, select products with the following natural sweeteners.

MALTED GRAIN SYRUPS

Malted grain syrups include brown rice syrup and barley malt syrup. These sweeteners are produced by the simple process of malting. When we chew grains, the enzyme amylase (in saliva) breaks down the starch into simple sugars. The malting process does the same thing because malt enzymes convert the starch in grains into sweet syrup. Malted grain syrups provide a slow but prolonged source of energy because they metabolize slowly and evenly in the body, creating none of the severe stress reactions, such as rapid fluctuations in blood sugar levels, seen with fructose, glucose and sucrose.

DATES AND DATE SUGAR

The sugar that comes from dates has not been refined and therefore has had limited processing. Unlike refined sugars, it has kept most of its fibre and nutritional properties.

COCONUT PALM SUGAR

Coconut palm sugar is the crystallized nectar of the tropical coconut palm tree blossom. When evaporated this nectar is crushed into a wonderful, raw, sun-kissed sweetener which isn't too sweet and has a hint of caramel in its flavour. It contains twelve amino acids, potassium, magnesium, phosphorous, iron and zinc. It can be used as a replacement for refined sugar in a 1:1 ratio.

PURE MAPLE SYRUP

Pure maple syrup is produced from the sap of the maple tree when spring arrives in various parts of North America. The sap has to be boiled to concentrate the sugars. It contains complex carbohydrates and trace minerals which makes it a healthier choice than refined sugar. Avoid maple-flavoured syrup which is not the same thing as pure maple syrup.

Honey

Many people think honey is a healthy form of sugar. For a number of reasons it is no longer considered to be a healthier option than processed sucrose. Honey raises blood sugar levels more than sucrose, having the highest sugar content of all natural sweeteners, being 70 per cent sweeter than sugar. The amount of minerals and vitamins in honey are so tiny they are virtually inconsequential, and the enzymes that are present when it is raw are destroyed by the heating manufacturers use when processing honey to enhance its visual appeal.

There are a few exceptions though, such as Manuka honey, which is unheated and contains high levels of anti-oxidants as well as other nutrients and enzymes. These unprocessed forms of honey are used as healing agents but they won't remove a desire for sweet foods and can still cause blood glucose instability.

The glycaemic index and calorie counting

The glycaemic index (GI) is the measure out of 100 of how quickly the carbohydrate in a food is released into your bloodstream. It's about whether the food is a fast- or slow-releasing food and measures this quality, not the nutritional content of the carbohydrate itself. A score of 100 is the highest score you can have and the lower the food score the better the food is supposed to be for you. However, high fructose foods often have low GI scores because fructose doesn't stimulate insulin production, yet excess fructose is not healthy. Furthermore, different people seem to respond differently to similar GI value foods.

Conversely, when looking at carbohydrate counting or what is also called 'calorie counting', this measure tells you how much of the food is carbohydrate, but doesn't tell you what it does to your blood sugar levels.

Putting these two measures together gives you the glycaemic load (GL), which looks at the quality AND quantity of the carbohydrates.

Following a chart for the rest of your life is a pretty daunting prospect and the inconsistencies between the various methods that have been developed to 'help' people assess the quality of a food are somewhat confusing. When something is too difficult, most people just give up trying to understand the concept and go back to eating the same old way.

Always keep in mind that natural, unprocessed carbohydrates that have had minimal interference from processing are always better for you, and that fresh seasonal produce full of fibre will keep your blood sugar levels stable as well as your mood, concentration, weight and energy.

Sweets should be an occasional treat

Sugar in any concentrated form is not conducive to optimal physical or mental wellbeing. Undernourished and over-sugared brains are unlikely to function optimally or provide stable moods and concentration capabilities. However, we all have an evolutionary desire for sweet foods because dense carbohydrates give us a quick boost or spurt of energy, which was of great help when we were starving.

It is therefore extremely useful to learn how to make sweet treats that are nutrient dense and support optimal brain function. The recipes in this book contain natural forms of sugar and are meant to be enjoyed as occasional treats. They are also full of other important nutrients, making them nutrient-dense treats.

Avoid AGEs to avoid ageing

Advanced glycation end products (AGEs) are compounds formed when proteins are exposed to sugars. They can come about in two ways. When foods that contain protein are cooked with sugar, the heat acts on the exposed molecules, changing their composition and turning them brown or 'caramelizing' them. Although this improves both the taste and look of the food (think of light golden cookies, browned bread crusts and potato crisps), it forms AGEs. The second way that AGEs are formed is when you eat refined sugars and they interact with protein in your body. AGEs are responsible for damage to the arteries and veins, which leads to less reliable supplies of oxygen, blood and therefore nutrients to the cells and organs, including the heart and brain. AGEs also cause inflammation in the brain, as neurons cannot function optimally when their nutrient supply is compromised. AGEs stimulate the production of free radicals, which cause an ongoing cascade of damage in the brain. There is research to suggest that AGEs may promote beta-amyloid production in the brain, which is linked to Alzheimer's disease.

Action plan

Five things to do that will introduce more unrefined carbohydrates to your diet are:

1. Replace all soda drinks with pure fruit juice and dilute all fruit juices with water. Start with sparkling water and gradually move towards natural, plain water.

2. Read the labels of processed foods that you buy regularly and find replacements and/or dilute the products you already have with other low-sugar varieties (for example, mix sugar-laden breakfast cereals with low- or no-sugar varieties, aiming to consume no-sugar varieties). This is a very effective way to remove a vast amount of sugar from your diet quickly.

3. Replace all white sugar in your diet with rice syrup, coconut sugar, date sugar or pure maple syrup and use these new products sparingly in recipes you make regularly. By making your own naturally sweetened treats, you are satisfying your sweet tooth with nutrient-dense food.

4. Replace white carbohydrates with whole, unrefined options, such as white rice with brown rice, white pasta with a non-grain gluten-free pasta and sweet potatoes (kumera) instead of white potatoes. Consider non-grain options, such as quinoa (a seed), to replace grain-based meals.

5. Ensure you enjoy a well-balanced breakfast every morning to set the stage for stable blood glucose levels throughout the day.

See the Resources section for more supportive information.

CHAPTER 7

The foundation fats for your brain

Whenever I give a talk and explain the importance of fat in the diet, with particular reference to its importance for the brain, most people are very surprised. It seems the healthy low-fat diet myth is really entrenched in our culture and is a very challenging myth to expose and then discredit.

Many people actually get angry when they realize they've been fooled about how critically important fat is to our health, especially our mental health. For example, most people are not aware that after water, fat is the most abundant substance found in the body and brain. As every organ in the body is surrounded by fat and every tissue contains fat and every single cell is surrounded by fat, it should be a fundamental component of your diet. However, that's not what we've been told for decades! We've been advised to cut our intake of fat, so that now low-fat or no-fat diets are part of our culture.

The aim of this chapter is to give you a clear understanding of why you should add a pure, balanced, organic, cold-pressed essential fatty acid (EFA) blend of fats and oils to your diet every day. It also explains why you should eat nuts and seeds and oily fruits

STRUCTURE OF A TYPICAL NEURON

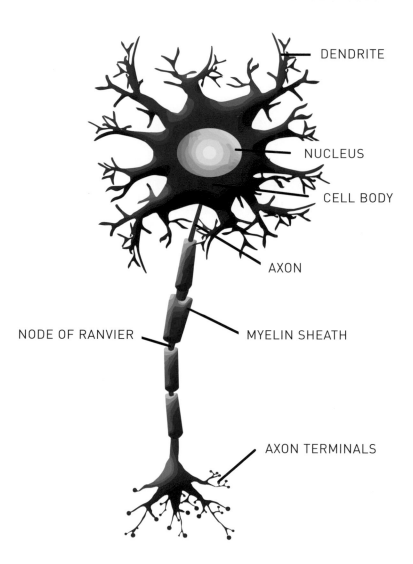

DENDRITE

NUCLEUS

CELL BODY

AXON

NODE OF RANVIER

MYELIN SHEATH

AXON TERMINALS

Although 20,000 neurons could fit onto the head of a pin, they are the greediest and most sophisticated cells we possess. They look like tiny trees with lots of branches and they use both electricity and chemicals to speak to each other.

such as olives and avocados daily and why you should replace shelf-stable vegetable oils and vegetable spreads with coconut oil, butter and olive oil.

Everyone's got a 'fat head'

Sixty per cent of the brain is made up of fat — yes, 60 per cent! That means that if you have been avoiding fat, chances are you suffer from low mood, possibly depression, and as you get older your ability to learn new things and to remember the skills you already have goes down drastically. In addition, you probably have sore joints, dry skin, dry eyes, a sluggish metabolism and low energy. Twenty-five per cent of that 60 per cent is made up of very specific types of fat, of which many people are unaware and therefore deficient in. Researchers now know that a lack of these specific types of fat is very likely to predispose you to memory decline, which in its drastic stages is also called Alzheimer's disease.

Professor Michael Crawford, the director of the Institute of Brain Chemistry and Human Nutrition at London Metropolitan University, has stated: 'Brain disorders and mental ill health have now overtaken all other burdens of ill health. The cost of mental ill health in the UK is £77 billion greater than heart disease and cancer combined. The impact on the next generation will be worse unless something is done. Therefore, the most important scientific question today is to reverse the climb in mental ill health and prevent brain disorders. We know that brain fats are a critically important part of the solution.'

Where is fat used in the brain?

Neurons are tiny specialized cells that help to make us who we are. There are a lot of neurons in the brain — about 100 billion. Furthermore, they are very tiny, with 20,000 of them being able to fit on the head of a pin. Each neuron is covered in a fatty membrane called a neuronal membrane and has tiny projections that stick out of it, called axons and dendrites, which are used to connect it to other neurons, so that they can communicate with one another. It has been calculated that a single neuron can make up to 20,000 connections with other neurons. The fatty neuronal membrane covers these tiny projections, which is where communication between these cells occurs. This is why the brain has such a large percentage of fat!

However, if the brain has the wrong kind of fat, then these cells will battle to talk to each other, which results in low mood, poor learning capacity and challenges with memory. If the brain has the right kind of fat, these cells will communicate with each other effectively and efficiently, keeping learning potential high and memory working optimally.

Some fats make membranes stiff and rigid, while others make them flexible and elastic. Obviously, the brain needs fats that allow these specialized membranes to be malleable — speed is of the essence in the brain, otherwise a thought will disappear. An example is when you walk into a room and can't remember why you are there! The thought got lost. Too many of those moments and you are in trouble.

Why the cell membrane is so important to neuron health

If the neuronal membrane does not have the right fats, it will be stiff and less pliable. This means that the neurons cannot have smooth conversations with each other, so the messages get muddled and don't get passed on correctly. It's like being on a very bad telephone line and trying desperately to hear what the other person is saying. If you cannot, you give up. This is what the neuron does too. The result is sluggish thinking, such as difficulty in learning a new task or recalling an old one, depression and anxiety, a lack of motivation, poor sleep and a lowered pain threshold. Interestingly, an impaired immune system and even body temperature imbalances also result. So, do unmotivated, unfocused and depressed people get sick more often? Yes. Research shows this is true!

The images overleaf are simplified illustrations of healthy versus unhealthy cell membranes. They show how important healthy cell membranes are in allowing nutrients and oxygen to flow into the cell and toxins to flow out.

How fast do your thoughts travel?

A special covering called myelin acts like an insulator along the special neuronal extension or axon. Myelin is very important because it helps to make sure the messages between neurons go at the right speed. I was amazed to discover that speeds of up to 350 kilometres per hour (220 miles per hour) can be reached between neurons — but only when the myelin contains, yes, you've guessed it, the right kinds of fat. If it is well formed, these speeds are maintained; when it is damaged or lacks the right fats, the speed slows.

An amazing 75 per cent of this myelin is made up of specialized fats, which is why a lack of them will definitely slow communication down between neurons. It has been estimated that if there is a deficiency in docosahexaenoic acid (DHA), the specialized omega-3 fatty acid that cold-water fish and algae contain, the signalling process between neurons can be slowed down by up to 90 per cent. Obviously, unmyelinated neurons or neurons with damaged or partial myelination will be unable to conduct nerve transmission effectively.

Furthermore, there are various illnesses, such as multiple sclerosis (MS), that can interfere with myelination with subsequent cognitive decline.

What does electricity do in your brain?

If you've heard that the brain runs on electricity, it's true! Thoughts travel through the neurons via electrical currents carried by neurotransmitters — the chemicals that work with electricity to make feelings and thoughts and generate actions. This is why these messages are called 'electro-chemical' impulses. Long strips of neurons light up with energy to form complete feelings, thoughts and memories.

The synapse is found at the end of axons and dendrites and is where neurons connect via neurotransmitters. The synapse has one of the highest concentrations of a specialized fat in the body and brain. If the synapse doesn't have the right kinds of fat present in its cells, it will not be able to release the neurotransmitter properly. So the messages between neurons will be garbled.

If any part of this electrochemical current is interrupted, the memory or thought becomes incomplete or is destroyed. That's partly what happens when you've walked into a room and forgotten why you went there in the first place.

So now you can see that brain function is based on the rapid transmission of electro-chemical impulses from one neuronal synapse to another, along the myelin sheath with

A HEALTHY VERSUS UNHEALTHY CELL MEMBRANE

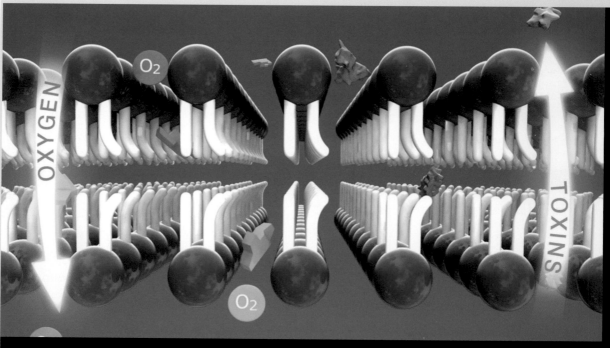

HEALTHY CELL

A healthy cell membrane is made up of fat molecules that are slightly 'curved' which give the membrane flexibility and the ability to interact with its contents and surroundings optimally. An unhealthy cell membrane is inflexible and hard, making it difficult to respond optimally to its contents and surroundings. Multiply these capacities by trillions of cells and you can imagine the impact healthy or unhealthy cell membranes have on your mental and physical health.

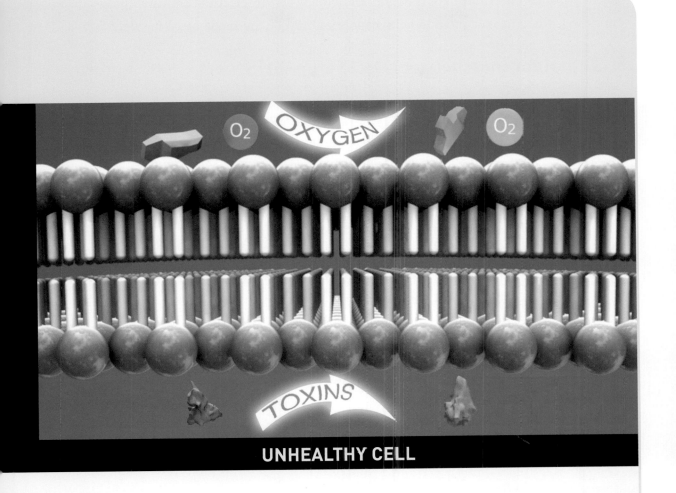

its fatty insulation. Amazingly, thoughts are actually all tiny electrochemical impulses that work well when the cell membrane, synapses and myelin are made up of the right fats.

The difference between fats and oils

The words fats and oils are used interchangeably, however they are not the same thing. Fats can become oils when they are heated but oils don't always become fats when they are cold or even frozen. For example, coconut oil turns solid when frozen and butter turns into a milky oil when it is heated. Some oils turn slightly solid when frozen, but quickly revert to being oils when brought to refrigerator temperatures. The different molecular properties of these compounds mean that they behave differently in your body as well. However, throughout this book, to make reading and understanding simple, I will refer to all the different kinds of fats and oils as just that: fats and oils.

What are the right kinds of fat for the brain?

The body can make both saturated fats and monounsaturated fats, but it cannot make a third type — polyunsaturated fats. The brain needs healthy forms of all these fats, especially polyunsaturated fats, to be able to work optimally. Because the body cannot make them, polyunsaturated fats are called essential fatty acids (EFAs) and have to be supplied by your diet. These fats ensure that cell membranes remain supple and flexible by providing them with a very high degree of elasticity and fluidity.

In addition, they ensure that inflammation is kept at a minimum in the brain, which is very important for optimal mental health.

Inflammation in the brain

Inflammation is a word derived from the Latin word *inflammatio* which means 'setting on fire'. Inflammation used to be associated with disease conditions that ended in 'itis' such as arthritis, but today we know that it is much more pervasive and involved in heart disease, obesity, diabetes and neuropsychiatric conditions. Inflammation is a state of unease and distress in the body, caused when cells aren't working optimally and are being either deprived of nutrients or are exposed to toxic substances such as pesticides, damaging fats and too many refined foods and additives. A lack of exercise and high levels of stress also add to a cell's inability to function well, and increase the chances of inflammation occurring. Inflammation of specialized cells, such as neurons, is a cause of great concern because mood, cognition and memory are all negatively impacted when this occurs. The brain is also extremely sensitive to physical injury, which can also cause severe inflammation and damage to brain cells. Cytokines are inflammatory chemicals produced in cell membranes when there is an excess of saturated fats, trans fats and too many omega-6 fats present in the diet. Inflammation can also lead to the breakdown of specific neurotransmitters such as serotonin, which is required to keep the brain working efficiently, especially with regards to mood maintenance and appetite regulation. Therefore the link between obesity, inflammation and depression comes as no surprise. The right essential fatty acids as well as a severe reduction or elimination of refined carbohydrates will ensure inflammation is kept at bay.

As the fats in the neuronal membrane are perpetually modelling and remodelling themselves in response to the messages they are constantly receiving, a lack of them will lead to less than optimal cognitive function. The brain never rests, so communication occurs 24/7. So, if you don't have the right kinds of fats available, these electrochemical signals cannot operate effectively.

There are two kinds of polyunsaturated fats in the neuronal membrane: omega-3 and omega-6 fatty acids. Most people know omega-3 fats as fish oils and believe that those are the only ones we need because the media has sold the message that we need to avoid all omega-6 oils. But this is not the whole story. Some omega-6 fatty acids are anti-inflammatory and some are inflammatory. The brain needs both omega-3 and omega-6 fats in an undamaged form and in the right ratio to function optimally, however most omega-6 fats found in supermarket products are damaged and toxic to human health.

To maintain a healthy brain, you need to understand how saturated fats, mono-unsaturated fats and polyunsaturated fats work.

Saturated fats

There are two kinds of saturated fats: plant forms of saturated fat and animal forms of saturated fats. If you didn't eat any saturated fats, your body could make them in the large intestine from sugars and starches, which is why they aren't 'essential'. In addition, the body converts excess saturated fats into monounsaturated fats to protect the body from the damage caused by excess saturated fats.

The plant forms of saturated fat contain medium-chain triglycerides (MCTs), which are absorbed directly into the bloodstream and used very efficiently for energy. They are solid at room temperature, contain large amounts of fatty acids (FAs) and include tropical fats such as coconut oil, palm kernel oil, cocoa butter and shea nut. Plant forms of saturated fat tend to be more beneficial for health than the saturated fats from animal products. This is due to the presence of MCTs, which are antimicrobial, antiparasitic, antifungal and increase metabolic activity. The MCTs in coconut are converted into ketones by the liver and can be used by the brain when glucose levels run low or when ageing results in impaired neuronal insulin functioning within the brain.

All animal products, such as meat and dairy products, contain saturated fats in the form of short-chain triglycerides and long-chain triglycerides. These fats harden membranes, leaving them inflexible and unable to respond quickly to the various jobs they have to do, which ultimately leads to sluggish thinking, forgetfulness and slower thought processing, as well as general cognitive decline. They can also impede the permeability of the cell membrane, which will negatively influence the membrane's ability to allow important substances into the cell and allow toxins out.

However, consuming enough EFAs naturally lessens these negative effects because the EFAs, being very soft and flexible, balance out the hardness and inflexibility of the saturated fats.

FLOWCHART OF
FATS AND OILS

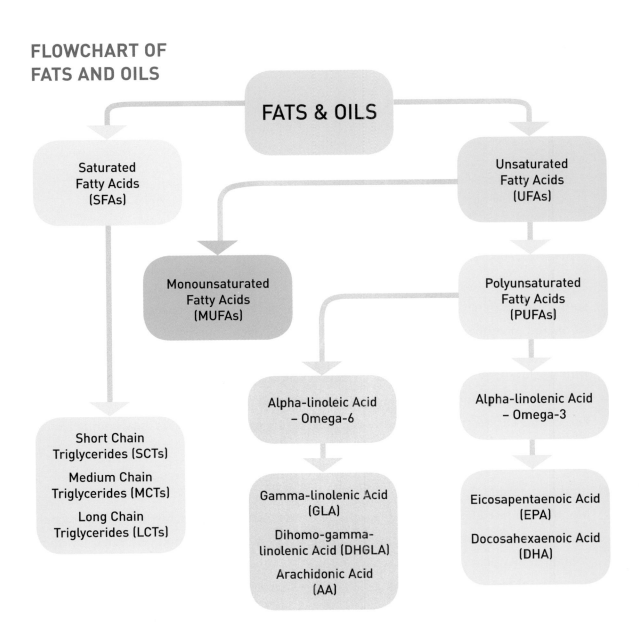

Fats and oils can be classified into two basic categories: saturated and unsaturated fats. These are then broken down into their respective groups: short-, medium- and long-chain saturated fats; monounsaturated (meaning 'one' double bond) fats; and polyunsaturated (meaning 'more than one' double bond) fats. Polyunsaturated fats are the only fats we cannot make and are therefore known as 'essential fats'.

Conjugated linoleic acid

Conjugated linoleic acid (CLA) is naturally synthesized from omega-6 fatty acids through a process called bacterial hydrogenation in the stomach of animals that chew the cud, such as cows and sheep. Naturally, the food products they provide us with, such as meat, milk, butter and cheese, contain CLA. CLA is produced when the omega-6 molecule moves one of its double bonds closer to the next one, producing a fat molecule that has double bonds two carbons apart rather than three carbons apart. In addition, one of the hydrogen atoms 'jumps' over to the other side of the fat molecule making it a trans fat molecule. CLA is a naturally made trans fat. Despite some positive research into its benefits, there is also evidence to suggest it may not be helpful. Either way, it is not an essential fatty acid and is therefore not required for optimal health.

Sources of saturated fats include animal products such as butter, cheese, yoghurt and the fat on and in animal flesh. Tropical plant foods such as coconut, palm kernel, shea nut and cocoa butter all contain saturated fats too. Saturated fats are the best kinds of fat to cook with because they are less prone to oxidation and less sensitive to heat. I realize this goes against general opinion, which suggests that olive oil or canola oil are best to cook with, but science has the final say. The molecular structure of the fat or oil is the deciding factor, not popular opinion.

Monounsaturated fats and oils

Monounsaturated fats and oils are used extensively today. Traditionally these oils are eaten in Mediterranean countries with olives being the best-known monounsaturated fat (they contain a fatty acid called oleic acid or omega-9). Monounsaturated fats and oils stay liquid at room temperature but will get slightly thicker when refrigerated. They have a neutral effect on blood cholesterol, although too much can raise triglycerides. The exception though is olive oil, which lowers cholesterol due to its natural, active components. These oils are healthy to use if they are true cold-pressed and extra-virgin oils. Be sure to check that they have not been adulterated with cheaper, solvent-extracted oils, as there is no international governing body to enforce rules and regulations on olive oil or any oils for human consumption. See the Resources section for more information on buying undamaged fats and oils.

Sources of monounsaturated fats include olives, avocados, almonds, hazelnuts, peanuts, macadamia nuts and pistachios. Although these great-tasting and healthy fats are available everywhere today, they are not essential. Furthermore, if we eat too many carbohydrates and don't exercise enough, the body, to protect itself from the toxic effects of excess carbohydrates, will turn them into saturated and also monounsaturated fats. It is important to note that omega-7 is also a monounsaturated fat. It is found in sea buckthorn berries, some fish and macadamia nuts. It is also a non-essential fat, so the body can make it from carbohydrates too.

Polyunsaturated fats and oils

Polyunsaturated fats and oils are really precious. Without them, no matter what other good nutrients you consume, your health will never be optimal. A large percentage of your brain is made up of these unique fats and without them your cognitive wellbeing will be adversely affected.

Polyunsaturated fats are generally known as oils because they are liquid at room temperature, although researchers call them fats. They are called essential fatty acids or EFAs because firstly, we cannot make them, and secondly because they have two or more double bonds between carbons.

Polyunsaturated fats can be divided into two categories: omega-3 and omega-6 fatty acids. The following section explains these two varieties of polyunsaturated fats and how they work in the body.

OMEGA-3 POLYUNSATURATED FATTY ACIDS (PUFAS)

Omega-3 fatty acids are found in both plant and animal foods and are made up of three types: alpha-linolenic acid (ALA), docosahexaenoic acid (DHA) and eicosapentaenoic acid (EPA). ALA is a short-chain omega-3 fatty acid, while DHA and EPA are long-chain omega-3 fatty acids. Omega-3 fatty acids are five times more sensitive to damage through light, oxygen and heat than omega-6s.

Omega-3 fatty acids are critically important for brain development and function because they are involved in neuronal membrane construction and functioning. They influence energy production within the neuron, the production of specific proteins within the neuronal membrane and reduce inflammation. They are associated with increased cerebral blood flow and the increased transport of glucose across the blood–brain barrier. They affect the signalling that occurs between neurons and boost the creation of new synapses and new neurons. These special fats also allow our cells to use oxygen efficiently, naturally increasing energy levels and improving cellular functioning. This explains the positive impact of omega-3 fats on immune function, blood pressure, endocrine function, blood glucose levels, mood, memory and learning and metabolic activity.

The short-chain omega-3 ALA is found in chia seeds, flaxseed and hemp seeds and green leafy vegetables. Although pumpkin, walnuts and soya beans also contain some of these omega-3 fatty acids, they have more omega-6 fatty acids so are classified in this category.

Derivatives of omega-3 known as docosahexaenoic acid (DHA) and eicosapentaenoic acid (EPA) are found in cold-water fish and in a particular form of red-brown algae called *Crypthecodinium cohnii*. Both DHA and EPA are 25 times more sensitive to damage than omega-6s.

Getting all your omega-3s

The body has the ability to take the omega fatty acids and turn them into derivatives. For example, DHA and EPA are both formed from the omega-3 alpha-linolenic acid (ALA) and GLA and AA are from the omega-6 linoleic acid (LA). The body needs specific nutrients such as vitamin C, vitamin B3 and vitamin B6, as well as the minerals magnesium and zinc to do this conversion with ease.

Cold-water fish such as salmon, mackerel and herring already contain the two derivatives DHA and EPA that the body can make from plant forms of omega-3 because they have eaten the algae that contains DHA and EPA. Many people also assume that the plant form of omega-3 is ALL converted into the derivatives DHA and EPA, which is not the case at all! Only 2–5 per cent of the base plant forms of omega-3 are converted into DHA or EPA, which leaves the remaining omega-3 to perform other essential tasks in the cell membrane and within the cell. So, if you only consume fish oil to get your omega-3s, you are only receiving a small percentage of the benefit of omega-3 and losing out on up to 98 per cent of the benefit that you could be receiving!

Unfortunately, due to a number of different factors, including the exceptional marketing skills of fish oil manufacturers, people now believe these are the only omega-3s they need to consume. This is one of the reasons the consumption of fish oil has become so prevalent. The generally recommended intake of DHA and EPA is 500–1000 mg per day, however, three capsules of fish oil generally provides only 360–540 mg. Adding 2 tablespoons of a plant-based omega-3 oil blend to your diet each day will ensure you get the recommended daily intake of DHA and EPA at the 2–5 per cent conversion rate, if your body can do the conversion efficiently.

OMEGA-6 POLYUNSATURATED FATTY ACIDS (PUFAS)

This group of oils is also called linoleic acid (LA). Sources rich in omega-6 include safflower seeds, sunflower seeds, sesame seeds, soya beans, corn, pumpkin and walnuts. Derivatives of omega-6 are gamma-linolenic acid or GLA (found in evening primrose oil and borage seed oil) and arachidonic acid or AA (found in animal products). They have not gained as much attention as the omega-3 derivatives DHA and EPA, but they also have very important roles to play in health and disease.

GLA prevents the blood platelets from sticking together, thereby averting blood clots in arteries. It is also responsible for relaxing blood vessels, lowering blood pressure and improving circulation. GLA is also very useful in preventing premenstrual syndrome (PMS) and can improve specific types of eczema too. It also stops the release of excess arachidonic acid from cell membranes, being in effect an anti-inflammatory agent.

Arachidonic acid, although responsible for some pro-inflammatory actions, is also very important for optimal brain function. AA is involved in the plasticity of neuronal synapses, which ensures memory consolidation and neurotransmitter release. It is also responsible for spatial learning. Due to the overconsumption of omega-6 fats and oils,

CATEGORIES OF FATS AND OILS
According to Majority Fatty Acid Content

*Most oils contain varying proportions of different fatty acids. ** Reacts different in body vs. animal saturated fats. *** May not be the healthy oil we've been told it is.*

SATURATED FATS AND OILS	UNSATURATED FATS AND OILS		
	Mono-unsaturated Fats and Oils	**Polyunsaturated Oils** **Omega-6** (Alpha-linoleic Acid) **Omega-3** (Alpha-linolenic Acid) (SUFA)	
		Omega-6 (A-linoleic Acid)	**Omega-3** (A-linolenic Acid)
Animal products • Butter, cream, cheese, etc. (contain SCT) • Meat – most kinds (contain LCT) **Tropical Plants**** • Cocoa butter • Coconut cream, milk and oil (contain MCT) • Palm kernel oil • Shea nut butter	• Almonds • Argan seeds (has high Omega-6 too) • Avocados • Brazil nuts • Cashew nuts • Hazelnus • Macadamia nuts • Neem nuts • Olives • Peanuts • Pecan nuts • Pistachio nuts	• Canola seeds*** • Corn • Cotton seeds • Grape seeds • Hemp seeds • Pumpkin seeds • Safflower seeds • Sesame seeds • Soya beans • Sunflower seeds • Walnuts GLA (Gamma-linolenic Acid) Evening Primrose seeds Borage seeds Blackcurrant seeds & AA (Arachidonic Acid) Prostaglandin (1 & 2) – H_2O balance; blood thickness and vessel relaxation; blood pressure decrease; decrease inflammation; increase immune and nerve function; assists insulin	• Chia seeds • Flax seeds • Dark green leafy vegetables EPA and DHA present in fatty fish (salmon, trout, sardines, mackerel, herring) Prostaglandin (3) – brain function; nerve cell membranes; vision; learning ability; co-ordination; mood; immune function; metabolism
		GLA (OM 6) ▶ DHGLA (Dihomo-gamma-linoleic Acid) ▶ AA (Arachidonic Acid)	
Only heat occasionally	Only heat occasionally	Never heat any of these oils	

The chart above simplifies fats and oils even further, providing examples of the types of foods where specific fats and oils are found. Polyunsaturated fats are the most complex because both of these special omega 'essential fats' get converted into important cell messengers, which perform many critically important functions in the brain and body.

and too many animal products, many people have too much arachidonic acid in their diet, which results in a general state of inflammation. In addition, without enough omega-3s, the balance is skewed in favor of omega-6. However, the consumption of undamaged omega-3 fats and oils will ensure that this balance is kept in check.

Mental health and EFAs

Mental illness is linked to a lack of essential fatty acids, and we all know that mental illness is alarmingly on the rise. Even skin disorders are more prevalent among people who do not eat any or enough of these important essential fats. And then there is the impact of stress — when you are stressed by external circumstances you need even more of these essential fatty acids, as stress depletes them quickly. So not having EFAs in your diet puts extra stress on your body and brain!

Some of the mechanisms that are thought to link mental illness to a lack of EFAs are as follows:

- Lack of DHA in the neuronal membranes may lead to the depletion of serotonin and dopamine levels by up to 50 per cent.
- Lack of EFAs impairs neuronal migration, connectivity and timed apoptosis (cell death) and contributes to dendritic problems which leads to irreversible interruptions in the neuronal pathways regulating behaviour.
- Neuroinflammatory processes as well as dysregulation of the HPA (hypothalamus-pituitary-adrenal) axis are affected by extremely low levels of EFAs which, in turn, increases stress levels and feelings of anxiety, which may lead to behavioural challenges.

We now know the body needs the base essential fats of omega-3 (alpha-linolenic acid or ALA) and omega-6 (linoleic acid or LA), as well as the derivatives DHA, EPA, GLA and AA to sustain optimum health. So, simply consuming fish oil won't provide you with all these other essential nutrients.

If you think you are deficient in these essential fatty acids, the simple solution is to see whether you regain your health when you consume the plant forms of omega-3 and omega-6. If after three to six months you don't feel significantly better, add an organic EFA blend that contains algae with the derivatives DHA and EPA and not fish oils, which are generally damaged through processing (see 'Fish oil supplements' on page 155). In addition, consume organic plant foods which contain these essential fats, such as crushed flax-seeds, soaked and crushed chia seeds and wild cold-water fish. Most healthy people can make enough of the derivatives from the foundation fats but some people cannot. See the resources section for recommended products.

For the best health outcomes, the ratio between omega-3 and omega-6 in the body needs to be 2:1 because omega-3s are involved in the function of highly biologically active organs like the brain, heart, reproductive organs and the adrenal glands, so they need to be available in greater quantities. Omega-6s are used in less active tissues.

EFAs and vision, hearing and taste

Vision, hearing and taste may all be influenced negatively by a deficiency in omega-3 fatty acids. As the retina is one of the tissues in the body that has the highest concentration of omega-3s, a deficiency induces changes in the membranes of the retina that are associated with an inability to detect light. Research has shown that the retina needs ten times more light to respond when it is deficient in EFAs. The cerebral response to auditory stimuli is also influenced by a deficiency in omega-3 fatty acids, as well as low levels of EFAs accelerating the ageing of the auditory system.

What else do essential fatty acids do?

Tiny compounds in the body called eicosanoids, which can also be called messengers or signalling agents because they carry messages or signals between the cells, are made from the all-important omega-3 and omega-6 fatty acids.

Eicosanoids are short-lived, hormone-like substances that regulate metabolism, anti-inflammatory actions, vision, learning ability, co-ordination, mood, brain function, immune function as well as body–water balance, blood vessel relaxation, blood pressure, nerve function and insulin function.

The eicosanoid group of compounds is a large family made up of many subgroups. Prostaglandins, lipoxins, leukotrienes and thromboxanes are some of them, and they each have different and very specific functions. Some of them are also stronger than others in their actions and functions. They play a balancing act with their roles and many aspects of their function are still to be discovered.

The eicosanoids that originate from DHA and EPA (omega-3 derivatives) are mildly anti-inflammatory and facilitate immune function. They have a critically important role to play in maintaining a healthy central nervous system, including the brain.

The eicosanoids that originate from GLA (an omega-6 derivative) are anti-inflammatory in nature, which means they stop inflammation and also improve immunity. They can also help with skin conditions such as eczema as well as depression, PMS and ADHD.

The eicosanoids that originate from AA (an omega-6 derivative) are actively involved in causing inflammation, which is necessary at particular times such as when the immune system needs to respond quickly when bleeding needs to stop and when pain signals are required.

But when eicosanoids are produced in excess due to the consumption of too many damaging omega-6 fatty acids, they cause a state of inflammation within the cells, tissues and organs, including the brain, which causes long-term damage and disease.

Essential fatty acids are very fussy

Essential fatty acids don't like to be exposed to light, heat, oxygen or moisture, therefore processing causes extreme damage to them. Damaged fats are also called oxidized fats because they have been exposed to oxygen, which causes damage to their delicate molecular structure. They then become toxic to cells, tissues and organs, causing distress and inflammation.

About two-thirds of dietary fats consumed today are omega-6 fatty acids of vegetable origin (for example sunflower, soya, corn or canola in the form of margarine or shortening). Most of these omega-6 fats have been exposed to the elements during harsh processing and are therefore damaged. When they are exposed to the elements their structure changes shape and they subsequently cannot perform their unique functions inside our cell membranes and cells.

Essential fatty acids become damaged through harsh processing methods that use chemicals to suck the oils out of EFA-containing seeds, as well as by heat to remove any compounds that would lead to less shelf-stable products. Fish oil is also subjected to harsh processing methods in an attempt to get rid of the mercury and other damaging compounds found in our oceans today. As a result, many products contain these damaged fats including margarines and fake butters, pastries, pies, sausage rolls, cakes and scones, muesli, granola bars and protein bars, potato chips and crackers, soups, frozen foods, baked goods, breakfast cereals, creams in cans, dips and salad dressings, cookies and candies/lollies and, of course, essential fat supplements.

When essential fats are damaged, the body doesn't really know what to do with them because they are still fats and will still go where essential fats are needed, but they cannot perform the duties of an undamaged essential fat. Their molecular shape isn't recognized within the cell membrane. Consequently, the damaged polyunsaturated fats and oils make cell membranes hard, inflexible and impermeable, exactly the opposite of what cell membranes should be. They are impostors unable to do the job and they take up the space where a good, undamaged essential fat should be.

Even though polyunsaturated EFAs are more sensitive to damage from the elements due to their more delicate molecular make-up, that does not mean that saturated and monounsaturated fats are immune to damage either. Although saturated fats can tolerate more heat than monounsaturated and polyunsaturated fats and oils, excess heat will still cause damage to the saturated fat molecules. Minimally processed, organic and cold-pressed fats and oils should be your choice if you desire optimum health. Organic butter, cold-pressed organic coconut oil, organic extra-virgin cold-pressed olive oil and organic essential fatty acid oil blends are best.

Fish oil supplements

When you read the words 'pharmaceutical quality' on the side of a fish oil supplement, you may not immediately think the product is highly refined. The term is misleading because it means the fish oil has been subjected to very high levels of heat in an attempt to get rid of toxic compounds via evaporation. Unfortunately, due to this exposure to very high temperatures, most fish oil supplements contain trans fats, fragmented fatty acids and polymerized fats. None of these damaged fats enhance your mental or physical health.

What about eating fish?

I remember as a child my parents telling me that fish was 'brain food'. Unfortunately, fish today are not the same as they were a few decades ago. As a planet, our supplies of fish are becoming ever more limited with scientific consensus having been reached on the rapid and unrelenting decline of worldwide fish stocks. There are over 100 confirmed cases of extinction of marine wildlife in the oceans of the world. Catches of wild Atlantic salmon have been in decline throughout the North Atlantic area since 1973. This species is now on the brink of extinction in the United States.

The causes for this devastating decline are many, all linked to human activity destroying their fragile ecosystem. Freshwater acidification caused by acid rain and chemical pollutants have impacted the feeding, growth and hormonal development of the fish; while dam construction, erosion and aquaculture, resulting in escaping salmon, has led to hybridization between the wild and farmed species. This, in turn, has resulted in the erosion of the genetic adaptation of salmon to local environments.

Fish farms and aquaculture are not long-term solutions as the fish that are being raised in these unnatural environments are mostly carnivorous so have to obtain their nutrition from smaller fish, which have been turned into fishmeal and fish oils.

Contaminants in fish are also problematic, with industrial waste being largely responsible for the toxins (such as PCBs, mercury and dioxins) that have accumulated in the fish. Worldwide, farmed salmon have been shown to have higher levels of some of these toxins than wild salmon. As a result, eating these fish gets these toxins into our brain.

The problem with farmed fish

Wild salmon eat krill that feed on red algae, which is why their flesh has a natural pinkish hue. Organically farmed salmon are fed natural shrimp shell, which they also consume in the wild, which also leads to their natural colour. However, conventionally farmed salmon are fed artificial dyes that act like beta-carotene and colour the flesh to increase their pinkness to quite a vivid hue.

Whether fish are farmed conventionally or organically, they are brought to market earlier than those caught in the wild. Fish farming is now the fastest growing food sector due to the collapse of ocean fish stocks. Farmed salmon does not always contain enough of the omega-3s required for so-called heart benefits and can contain 15 per cent less protein than their wild counterparts. Farmed salmon also contain up to 10 times the PCBs and dioxins when compared to wild salmon and it's believed that the source of these toxins is the fish oil and fish meal they are fed. Farmed salmon are also exposed to vast quantities of antibiotics, anti-fungal agents and other potentially harmful compounds.

Exposure to mercury has been shown to cause neurological damage, as well as damage to the liver and kidneys. Mercury has a special affinity to fat because it is soluble in fat, so the heavy metal automatically migrates to fat cells and cell membranes. With our brain being 60 per cent fat, this is of particular concern.

Some countries such as Canada have issued regulations regarding consumer consumption of predatory fish due to mercury, but no such directive has been issued with regards to PCB or dioxin exposure from contaminated fish. And although there are researchers who believe the benefits of consuming fish outweigh the potential risks, please remember that we are not producing less toxic waste each year, but more.

The evaluation of the risk has to be an ongoing process and it's not possible for that to occur on a global scale and for the consumer to be kept up to date. Try to ensure that the fish you eat is free of contaminants, although this is becoming less and less feasible.

Generally speaking, small, deep-sea fish such as anchovies and sardines are less exposed to toxic contamination, simply due to their size and shorter life spans. However, ocean toxicity is not decreasing so be sure that you are not relying on fish alone to give you the important EFAs you need.

What about cholesterol?

Cholesterol is a hard, crystalline substance technically classified as a steroid. However, it is soluble in fat rather than water, so is also classified as a lipid or fat. Cholesterol has received a lot of bad press and most people don't understand the important role it plays in our physical and mental wellbeing. It is found naturally in the brain, nerves, liver, blood and bile of humans.

The liver manufactures about 80 per cent of the body's cholesterol, whereas 20 per cent comes from the diet. About half of the cholesterol that we consume from our diet is absorbed and the other half passes through our bodies unused. In about 70 per cent of people, the feedback loop that lowers cholesterol production within our bodies when our dietary intake is excessive is very effective; the other 30 per cent have a defective feedback loop and they can suffer from excess cholesterol if their diet is not managed and they eat too many animal products.

Here are few of the important things that cholesterol does, influencing both our mental and physical wellbeing:

- Cholesterol ensures the fluidity of our cell membranes. If our cell membranes get too hard, they can't work properly and if they get too soft, the same thing happens. Cholesterol cannot do its job optimally if there are not enough of the right EFAs in the cell membrane.

- Serotonin, which is both a hormone and a neurotransmitter, induces a sense of calm and suppresses feelings of aggression. Low cholesterol levels reduce the amount of serotonin receptors on our neuronal membranes, thereby contributing to feelings of anxiety, irritability, aggression and hostility.

- Cholesterol helps to make the sex hormones progesterone, estrogen and testosterone.

- Cholesterol makes adrenal corticosteroid hormones, which are the hormones produced when we are stressed, scared or anxious. The best-known is adrenaline which later becomes cortisol. This, in turn, stimulates the production of glucose to help with the stress response.

- Cholesterol is responsible for the production of vitamin D, which occurs as a result of the sun's action on the skin, ensuring healthy bones, a healthy immune system and optimally functioning hormones.

Good and bad cholesterol

Lipoproteins help cholesterol travel from the liver to various tissues in the body. The cells use what they need and any extra remains in the bloodstream until other lipoproteins pick it up for transport back to the liver. Low-density lipoproteins or LDLs are considered 'bad' cholesterol because they are laden with the substance, whereas high-density lipoproteins or HDLs are 'good' because they circulate in the bloodstream picking up excess cholesterol from blood and tissues. If everything is functioning well, this system works with the LDLs bringing the cholesterol to the cells and the HDLs picking up the 'leftovers' and taking them back to the liver to be used again by the LDLs. But if there's too much for the HDLs to pick up quickly, then cholesterol may become the plaque that damages artery walls, leading to heart disease. To keep a balance in the body's cholesterol levels you need to avoid eating processed foods with damaging fats in them and refined sugar, which also increases cholesterol production. Essential fatty acids from whole foods and leafy greens also help to maintain this balance. Keep in mind that stress also forces your body to produce cholesterol.

How much EFAs do you need every day?

Your diet should favour omega-3s because they are used in the most metabolically active organs, such the brain, heart, hormone system and adrenal glands. The ratio of two parts omega-3 to one part omega-6 (2:1) may be the best way to get your omega-3 deficiency solved while still supplying the important omega-6s. Of course, avoiding all shelf-stable, processed frying oils is also an important step in the process of replenishing your cells with the right fats and getting rid of the damaging ones.

However, if you are very deficient in omega-3 oils, which most people are, you can start by eating only cold-pressed, organic flaxseed oil for a few months and later add cold-pressed omega-6 oils like sunflower or sesame seed oils to the mix. But remember that the ratio should be 2:1 in favour of omega-3. If your symptoms do not significantly improve, then you can add a DHA and EPA supplement to the basic foundation fats you are eating, as you may not be able to do the conversion from the plant-based flaxseed oil to the derivatives DHA and EPA, as discussed on page 152.

There are a number of symptoms that indicate a deficiency in essential fatty acids. The skin, being such a large organ, will generally show symptoms of deficiency first. If you experience more than five of the symptoms below, the chances are very high that you suffer from either an imbalance or a deficiency of EFAs or both:

- dry skin and/or skin rashes (including acne)
- excessive thirst
- frequent urination
- cracked heels
- brittle hair
- dandruff
- brittle nails
- follicular hyperkeratosis or 'chicken skin' where the pores on the back of the arms and upper outside of the thighs become hard and dry, often filled with sebum
- mental challenges such as slow thinking, memory and attention difficulties
- problems with movement, balance, sensation or physical feeling
- feeling highly emotional
- unable to effectively handle relationships and interactions with others
- feelings of depression

- anxiety

- insomnia

- lack of physical energy

- sore joints

- sluggish metabolism

- hormonal imbalances.

There is research to indicate that introducing omega-3 (and undamaged omega-6) to your diet can rejuvenate your cell membranes within days. This is simply due to the fact that your cells have been craving these EFAs and put them to use immediately.

However, if many of the membranes of your cells are composed of damaging trans fats, it can take between eighteen months and three years to replace them all with the right kind of fats. Furthermore, the body will start using them where they are needed the most in the hardest working organs such as the brain, heart, hormonal system and adrenal glands.

Do fats and oils have to be organic?

All the foods that you choose to eat should ideally be organic because pesticides obviously do not support optimal health. However, many pesticides are oil-soluble which means that oily nuts and seeds will contain pesticide residues if they are not grown organically. Pesticides accumulate in the fat tissues of animals, including humans. This means that our cells and tissues will end up containing pesticides if we don't eat organic nuts, seeds and oils. As your brain is 60 per cent fat you don't want to take the chance of accumulating pesticides there!

Even if the oil you consume uses conventional seeds that have had the pesticides removed, the process of removing these chemicals is accomplished through deodorization. This harsh process only removes half of the pesticides, leaving the oil damaged as well as producing other toxic substances.

Cooking with fats and oils

Cooking with fats and oils can be done healthily; just remember, the more saturated the fat, the safer it is to cook with.

A high heat (up to 190°C/374°F), such as used in frying, is best for saturated fats because they remain stable. These include coconut oil, palm kernel oil and cocoa butter. Butter is also a better choice than monounsaturated and polyunsaturated fats and oils. However, frying is not recommended for butter, as such high temperatures can still result in some fat (and food) becoming damaged.

Although plant forms of saturated fats are healthy and a better choice to cook with, they aren't if they have been damaged by processing. Coconut oil may be processed in similar ways to other shelf-stable fats and oils and is also often hydrogenated, leading to further damage and the addition of trans fats. When coconuts are exposed to light and oxygen for extended periods of time, they will become damaged. So use unrefined, tropical oils or, even better, eat the flesh of fresh coconuts.

Moderate heat (up to 170°C/338°F), such as used in sautéing and stir-frying, is best for monounsaturated fats and oils which don't contain EFAs. These oils are olive, almond, hazelnut, peanut and pistachio.

Low heat (less than 100°C/212°F), such as used in baking and making sauces, is best for polyunsaturated fats and oil. Safflower, sunflower and sesame oils are the ones to use. Baking bread and cakes at around 160°C (320°F) keeps the inside temperature of the food under 100°C (212°F), however the outside of the baked goods will contain damaged fats.

Use flax, hemp, pumpkin (pepita), walnut, sunflower and sesame seed oils that are cold pressed to prepare salad dressings, pestos, relishes, dips and mayonnaise. Due to their sensitivity to light, heat and oxygen they should never be heated. These oils contain omega-3 and omega-6 fatty acids.

Traditional cooks used fats and oils differently in their cooking than how the younger generations do now. Italians didn't throw olive oil over all their food before cooking it, or fry everything, as is now the case, since many cooking shows don't depict the reality of traditionally prepared food. Italians had a finite amount of oil to use for the year after harvesting. Chinese cooks traditionally added water to their woks and later added oil, which kept the oil temperature down and allowed the minimum use of oil.

Action plan

Five things to do that will introduce the right brain fats to your diet are:

1. Purchase and start using the best organic, unrefined essential fatty acid (EFA) supplement you can find.

2. Replace cooking oil with organic coconut oil and organic, grass-fed butter (in small quantities) and don't buy any more damaged, shelf-stable, vegetable oils.

3. Replace margarines and other vegetable spreads and oils with organic, unrefined oils such as olive oil, avocado, macadamia nut butter, tahini (sesame seed paste) and real butter.

4. Dry-bake potatoes and vegetables in the oven on silicon trays to stop sticking. Add oil, herbal salt, spices and herbs after baking for flavour.

5. Buy a variety of fresh nuts and seeds and keep them refrigerated, using them in salads, to make muesli (granola) bars and as great snacks.

See the Resources section for more information.

CHAPTER 8

A lighter, brighter you — putting it all together in 7 steps

Having some understanding of human nature and the consolidation of new habits due to my psychology background, my aim in writing this book was to make the information as simple as possible without losing the essence of the science. When you 'get' what I'm talking about, you are more eager to listen further and investigate the subject in more depth.

When starting out on the steps in this book, I want you to be able to commit to the first change that you decide to make for as long as it takes you to get it into your daily routine. If that takes a week, great; if it takes a month, that's fine too. The aim is to move steadily through the various steps until they are all a natural part of your daily life and you don't have to work at remembering them any more. That's how good habits 'stick' and change your life. For example, you may decide to start walking every day and remove sugary, processed foods from your diet. Stick with these two new habits until you don't have to think about them anymore and then move onto another step. I encourage you to move through all the steps to get the full benefit of their combined power. Adopting all the 7 steps will give you the greatest benefit.

Naturally, your brain will benefit from each of the steps as you implement the suggestions. Each change will automatically become simpler and easier because your brain will be functioning better. By providing your brain with the nutrients it needs to support you, you naturally start making better decisions about your health habits and the foods that you choose to eat. On top of this, you will notice many other great side effects. Your mood will naturally improve, which will lead to stable blood glucose levels. You will have fewer, if any, cravings, so your weight will start to stabilize and you will lose weight if you need to. Your memory, concentration and capacity to learn and remember new things will also improve because your brain will have the energy to facilitate these cognitive processes more efficiently. You will make better decisions and enjoy the results of those decisions.

It is so much easier to embark on a new way of eating if you have some basic recipes to nudge you onto the right path. Recipes that are tasty and super-quick to make will entice you to make positive changes. The next section of this book contains my 'go to' recipes — the ones that I rely on and make regularly to ensure good brain health. You will find various 'tweaks' at the end of most of the recipes, as I love to add new ingredients and change the flavour of dishes with ease. Also, as I rely on seasonal produce, I make changes as required too. I hope that you enjoy adding them to your new way of eating and that you soon find your favourites and healthily tweak them according to your personal preferences and what is in season in your part of the world!

I encourage you to remain committed to feeding your brain optimally because the positive cascade of benefits that you will enjoy will astound you. When you feed your brain optimally, you don't have to follow any other diet or eating plan. This is it — simple and straightforward. Deprivation and time-consuming commitments are discouraged because any new enterprise that requires these constraints generally fails. This is why you will find my recipes tasty and super-fast — and they include chocolate! The 7 steps in this book coupled with the recipes are designed to help you feed your brain to become a lighter, brighter you! Enjoy the experience.

Please go to www.lighterbrighteryou.life
**for more resources to support you
on your adventure.**

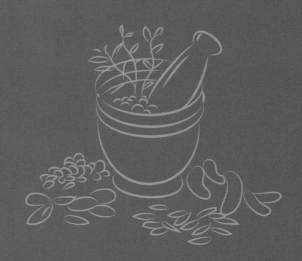

basic recipes for brain health

Introduction

Food should be healthy, nourishing AND tasty. When healthy food doesn't taste great, it is harder to stay committed to eating it. The brain enjoys novelty and stimulation, so bland and boring food leaves one craving tastier and more exciting food. Combining tasty, nutrient-dense foods with health in mind — specifically brain health — is the challenge that I faced when I learned what the brain needs to be optimally healthy. Visual appeal, taste and smell had to be taken into account because our sense organs play an important role in our appreciation and enjoyment of food.

This section presents a few of my favourite recipes — favourites because they are really quick and simple to prepare, and because I can mix and match various aspects of the dishes to make new meals and new tastes.

You will notice that all of the recipes use foods that contain fats and oils. As you will now know after reading Chapter 7, the brain loves fats and oils but they must be organic, pure and undamaged. In addition, flavour molecules disperse more efficiently in fats and oils than in water, so you have the added benefit of gaining tastier food when you add the right kinds of fats and oils to your meals. You will also notice that I do not fry many foods and if I do, I only use coconut oil.

Most of the recipes are colourful — the natural colours in food provide important nutrients. Of course, colourful food is also more appealing to your brain via your eyes, which increases your salivary response and gets digestive enzymes ready to help your body turn your food into fabulous fuel for your busy brain and body!

I also choose to use activated nuts, which are nuts with a brown skin that have been soaked for a number of hours or overnight to get rid of the enzyme-inhibitors that exist in their skin. They are then rinsed well and dehydrated in either a dehydrator or an oven at a very low temperature, such as 45–60°C (113–140°F). Therefore, when you read a recipe that calls for a nut that has a brown skin, assume that I mean it has been activated already. Nuts without a brown skin, such as cashew nuts or macadamia nuts, do not contain enzyme inhibitors, however they can be soaked in water to make them more digestible.

Please keep in mind that when cooking with real food there is variation in the quality and taste of the fresh produce. You may need to add a little more oil or some extra lemon juice to salad dressings, or some extra water when making nut creams. Cooking with real food means that you may have to be innovative at times and adjust as you go along. This is one of the reasons it is hard for people to cook with real foods when they have become used to cooking with packaged goods, highly flavoured sauces and preserved foods. These foods are designed to always deliver the same taste experience each time. Eating and preparing real food sometimes requires a touch of creativity.

As you start nourishing yourself with these real foods you will notice a subtle change in your taste buds and your body will start feeling satisfied earlier on in your meal. Your moods will become more stable, your memory will improve and you will start losing weight. This is to be expected when your brain starts receiving the nutrients that it craves for optimal functioning. Enjoy the experience!

Feel free to be flexible

It's important that you have fun preparing your food. Don't stress if you can't always find the fruit or nut specified in a recipe — choose another and experiment. You'll see in the recipe photographs that I often sprinkle extra nuts on my dishes, as I love the added crunch. Feel free to do the same ... or not! Now that you understand the 7 steps to brain health, this is your chance to make my recipes your own.

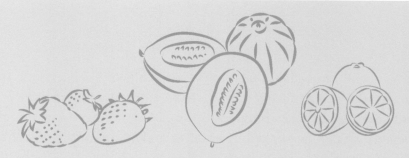

Breakfast

The recipes in this section are all sweet because most savoury breakfasts are really simple to prepare and need no explanation. You can make a wide variety of breakfasts using the Brain Breakfast Cereal recipe (pages 172–173) as a foundation. The same applies to the fruit smoothie recipes, which you can adapt and modify to your liking. Remember that breakfast is a very important meal and even if you are not hungry when you first wake up, which is normal, make sure that you have a healthy, brain-friendly meal at hand when you do feel the need to break your fast. Many cultures eat the same kind of food for breakfast as the rest of their meals. I eat salads, avocados and hummus for breakfast too! If you prefer a savoury breakfast, keep in mind that adding the right fats is very important.

Whether I am having a smoothie or a savoury breakfast, I always add an oil blend every morning (I use Udo's 3–6–9 Oil Blend). I stir it into my smoothie just before eating it, although you can easily add it to your smoothie before blending. If I'm eating a savoury breakfast, I drizzle it over my vegetables and leaves so that it combines well with all my food. After reading Chapter 7 you will now be very aware of how important it is to consume the right fats at meal times and breakfast is no exception! Your brain needs a steady supply of these special fats to stay healthy and vibrant and breakfast is a great opportunity to supply them daily!

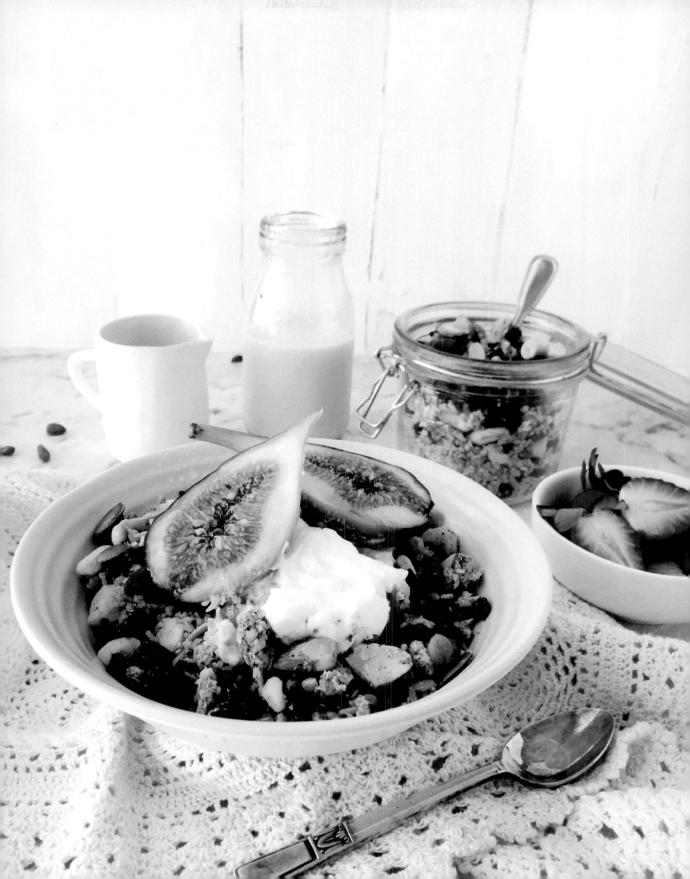

Brain Breakfast Cereal

MAKES 25–30 SERVINGS

This may seem like a lot of cereal but, believe me, it will disappear quickly. Making your own breakfast cereal means that you have control over what's in it! I add raisins, currants and finely chopped dried apples, dried apricots, dried cherries or dried blueberries to the mixture after it comes out of the oven. As this cereal contains some nuts and seeds, which contain essential brain fats, I called it the Brain Breakfast Cereal.

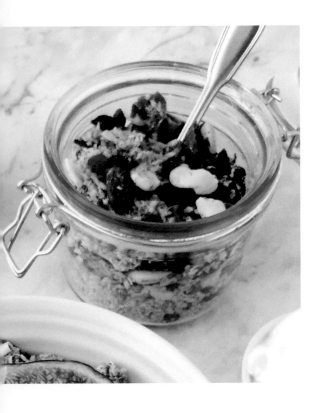

1½ cups amaranth flakes

1½ cups millet flakes

1½ cups quinoa flakes

1 cup desiccated coconut or coconut flakes

1 cup sunflower seeds

1 cup sesame seeds

1 cup walnuts

1 cup almonds

1 cup cashew nuts

1 cup pecan nuts

1 cup Brazil nuts

1 cup macadamia nuts

1 cup pumpkin seeds (pepitas)

1 cup olive or coconut oil

1 teaspoon pure vanilla essence (vanilla extract)

½ cup apple concentrate, brown rice syrup or pure maple syrup

zest of 2 organic oranges

1 teaspoon all spice

3 teaspoons cinnamon

2 cups raisins (or dried apple, dried cherries, dried apricots, dried blueberries, dried pineapple or dried mango finely chopped)

Preheat the oven to 50°C (122°F).

Mix the amaranth, millet and quinoa flakes with the coconut, sunflower and sesame seeds in a large bowl.

Coarsely chop the nuts in a food processor and add them to the large bowl with the gluten-free grains, coconut and seeds.

In a separate bowl, combine the olive or coconut oil with the vanilla essence, apple concentrate, orange zest, all spice and cinnamon.

Mix all the ingredients together, except the dried fruits, which you add after baking.

Spread the cereal on oven trays lined with baking paper and bake in the oven overnight until dry and crunchy.

Stir the mixture a few times before heading off to bed, and while still warm mix in your dried fruit of choice.

Cool and store in the refrigerator in a glass container with an airtight lid.

Variations

- Use 5½ cups oats in place of the gluten-free flakes if you can tolerate oats.

- If you just want muesli, leave out the oil, concentrate and zest and simply combine all the other ingredients.

- If you want to make the cereal a little more exotic, simply add 2–3 tablespoons of raw cacao powder or carob powder before you bake it in the oven. Add ¼ cup raw cacao nibs to the mixture when it comes out of the oven with the dried fruit of your choice.

NOTE

You can bake this cereal during the day if you start in the morning and stir it every few hours, removing it from the oven when dry and crunchy.

For a super-quick breakfast, ladle fresh berries into a glass, top with a dollop of either coconut yoghurt, Cashew Nut Cream or Macadamia Nut Cream (see Macadamia Mayonnaise recipe on page 193), then add a layer of the breakfast cereal. You can sprinkle a variety of nuts or seeds over the top of the cream too just to give it an extra nutrient boost. You can easily vary this breakfast according to the fruit in season — my favourite is combining fresh mango with fresh cherries.

Gluten–free Muffins

MAKES ABOUT 12 MUFFINS

These muffins are really simple to make and you can easily whip up a batch on a lazy weekend morning. I sometimes prepare all the ingredients the night before and surprise my family on a weekday morning. You can use 2 eggs instead of the polenta and psyllium husks, but reduce the coconut milk by 3 tablespoons, and the dried fruit can be substituted with some chopped nuts. Leave the muffins in the tins for about 20 minutes before removing them so that they can become a little firmer. Like all fresh preservative-free, gluten-free baked goods, these muffins are best on the day they are made.

Coconut oil

1 cup almond or hazelnut meal

1 cup Gluten-free Flour (see recipe on page 239)

2 teaspoons gluten-free baking powder

1 teaspoon ground cinnamon

1 tablespoon polenta

1 tablespoon psyllium husks

½ cup coconut oil (see Note)

¼ cup pure maple syrup or coconut nectar

1 teaspoon pure vanilla essence (vanilla extract)

2 medium bananas

1 cup coconut milk, at room temperature

Preheat the oven to 170°C (340°F).

Lightly oil a 12-hole muffin tray with coconut oil.

In a large mixing bowl, mix the almond or hazelnut meal, flour, baking powder and cinnamon until thoroughly combined.

In a separate bowl, add the polenta, psyllium husks, coconut oil, maple syrup, vanilla, bananas and coconut milk and mix until thoroughly combined.

Pour the wet ingredients into the flour mixture, add any extra ingredients of your choice such as dried fruit or chopped nuts, and stir until well combined. The liquid should be well absorbed but don't over-stir the mixture as it will get 'gluggy' because of the psyllium husks.

Evenly distribute the mixture into the muffin holes filling them up to the rim and bake for about 18–20 minutes until the muffins are lightly golden.

Variations

You can add about ¼ cup of any of these options, sprinkled on top of the muffins (or stirred through just before baking):

- finely chopped dried organic apricots
- coarsely chopped pecans, Brazil nuts, almonds, walnuts or pistachios
- 20 pitted fresh cherries
- fresh or frozen blueberries, raspberries or strawberries simply dropped onto the muffins before you bake them
- 10 chopped dates
- raisins, currants, sultanas
- 1 fresh chopped banana
- chocolate chips, to taste
- sprinkle of ground cinnamon, ground nutmeg or ginger to make them spicy
- sprinkle of coconut sugar.

You can also spread macadamia or almond nut butter over your muffin to increase its nutrient density and provide great fats and protein for your brain.

Note

If the coconut oil is solid, simply melt it in a small saucepan over a low heat until it is liquid.

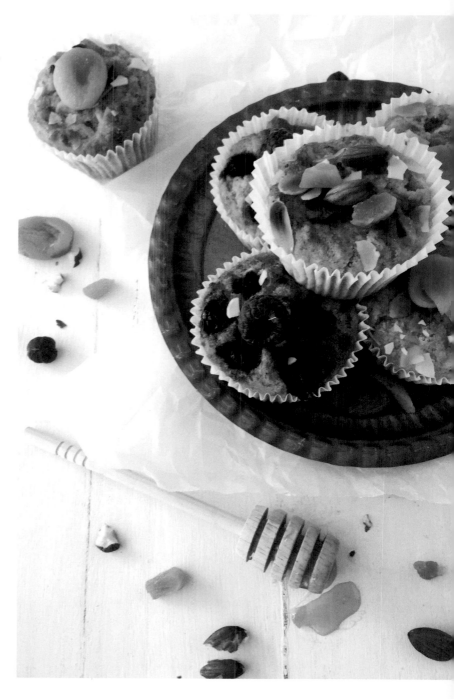

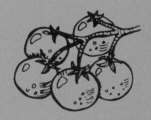

Fruit smoothies

Fruit smoothies are the simplest and tastiest breakfasts to make. I enjoy them year-round using various fruits in season. Experiment with what your family enjoys and see how simple breakfast can become. I love mango smoothies and freeze the flesh when a friend's trees generously supply them with extras! You can, of course, freeze any fruit and use them whenever you feel like making a smoothie. Adjust the amount of nuts and fruit according to how many people you plan to serve.

I generally use ¼ cup nuts, 1–2 cups fruit, 1 ice cube and ¼ cup liquid per person. You can also add a teaspoon of hemp protein powder per person. The variations are endless. And you can add any type of green leaves too, to increase the nutrient content!

Optimal digestion and absorption requires chewing, which adds specific enzymes to the foods in your mouth before you swallow the food. When a smoothie is too 'smooth' it doesn't require any chewing, so all those fabulous nutrients can end up in your digestive tract really quickly without the enzymes, unable to provide their full benefit. Therefore I always add a 'crunch' factor to my smoothies, so they are chewed instead of gulped down. An added advantage is that your brain starts to register satiation as you are filling up, rather than after you are too full.

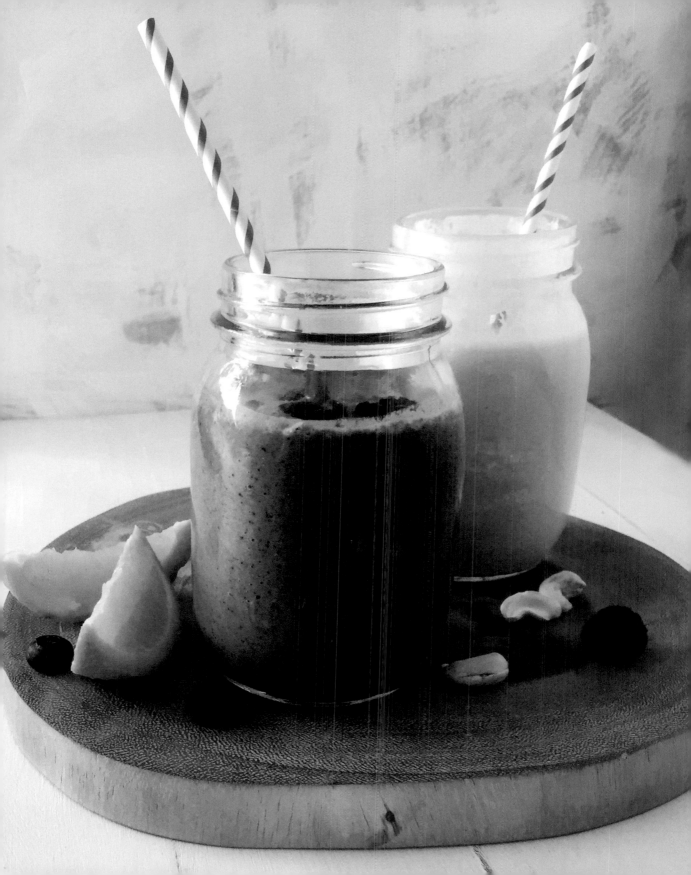

Mocha Smoothie

SERVES 4

This smoothie tastes more like a dessert than a breakfast! It's decadent but nutritious — the best combination!

2 bananas, frozen if possible

½ tablespoon coffee replacement or organic Swiss water-filtered decaffeinated coffee granules (see Notes)

½ tablespoon raw cacao powder

1½ cups coconut, rice or almond milk

½ cup cashew nuts

½ teaspoon pure vanilla essence (vanilla extract)

1 tablespoon coconut oil

1 medjool date, pitted

Combine all the ingredients in a blender until smooth and creamy.

Variations

- Add 1 scoop of hemp protein powder before blending for a complete meal.
- Almonds or macadamia nuts can be used as a replacement for the cashew nuts.
- Feel free to add a kale leaf or two — you can't taste them as the mocha flavour overpowers them.
- Sprinkle over raw cacao nibs for added crunch and flavour.
- Add 1 tablespoon hazelnut or peanut butter for a different flavour and added nutrients.

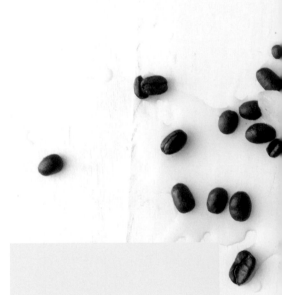

Notes

It is possible to find organic Swiss-water filtered decaffeinated coffee granules in some large stores now or you can use a coffee substitute.

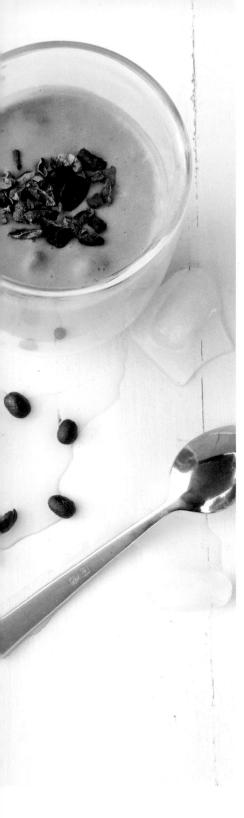

Breakfast Berry and Nut Smoothie

SERVES 4

This smoothie is thick and very fruity, so feel free to add coconut water to achieve the consistency you enjoy.

1 cup raw nuts (almonds or cashew nuts work well)

2 cups frozen mixed berries (strawberries, blackberries, blueberries, raspberries, cranberries)

1 cup pomegranate juice

2 oranges or mandarins

coconut water, according to taste

shaved coconut, hemp seeds, chia seeds, extra chopped almonds or pomegranate seeds, to taste

Combine the nuts, berries, pomegranate juice, oranges and coconut water in a blender until smooth.

Pour the mixture into a tall glass and top with shaved coconut, hemp seeds, chia seeds, chopped almonds or pomegranate seeds to add 'crunch'.

Eat the smoothie slowly with a spoon to savour the sublime rich, smooth flavour and texture.

Notes

Making a batch of coconut milk or coconut water ice cubes means that you can use them when making smoothies and end up with a super-cool and frothy drink. Simply freeze the coconut milk or coconut water in ice block trays, tip them out into a big glass container and keep them in the freezer for when you need them. You can do the same thing with lemon juice (for salad dressings) and other fruit juices, such as pomegranate juice.

Pineapple and Orange Smoothie

SERVES 4

This is a piña colada breakfast! If you don't have any frozen pineapple, simply add a few ice cubes to the mixture to keep it cool.

1 cup macadamia or cashew nuts

1 frozen pineapple, peeled, cored and cut into chunks

2 cups coconut milk or coconut cream

2 oranges, peeled

shaved coconut, hemp seeds, chia seeds or chopped almonds, to taste

Combine the nuts, pineapple, coconut milk or cream and oranges in a blender until smooth.

Pour the mixture into a tall glass and top with shaved coconut, hemp seeds, chia seeds or almonds to add 'crunch'.

Variations

- Replace the pineapple and oranges with 4 cups of fresh strawberries for a gorgeous pink, frothy smoothie.

- Replace the oranges with mandarins or tangelos for an equally delicious smoothie.

- Replace all the fruit with frozen cherries and the coconut milk with pomegranate juice.

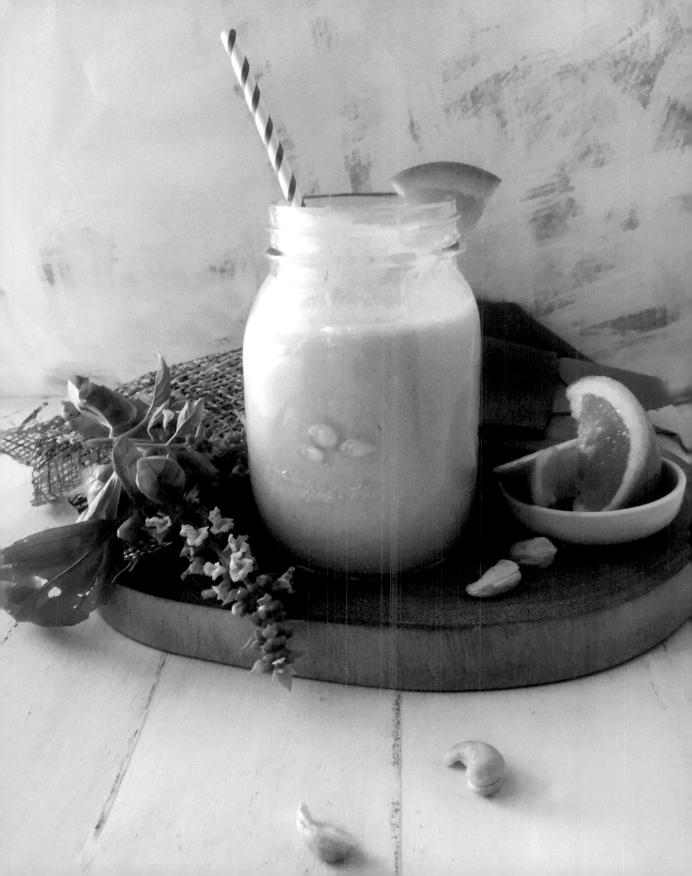

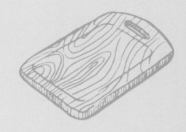

Snacks

The snacks in this section all contain a combination of protein, carbohydrates and fats to ensure even blood glucose levels and to satisfy our natural desire for something sweet. As they still contain a fair amount of sweetness, do not eat vast quantities of these foods — they are meant to satisfy a quick need for energy and not replace a whole meal! They can also be served as a dessert but keep in mind that the chocolatey ones should be reserved for a daytime snack as the theobromine in chocolate can keep sleep away!

Raw Date and Coconut Fudge

MAKES ABOUT 20 SLICES

This recipe is the result of a mistake I made one day while trying to combine dates and coconut to make a coarse, sweet mixture. I left the blender on while I attended to another task and when I looked next I'd turned the mixture into a ball of 'fudge'. It was a little warm so I simply pressed the whole mixture into a shallow dish, put it into the fridge and went into town. When I got back, I opened the fridge to discover a simple mistake had resulted in a splendid treat, one which we have enjoyed as a family ever since and which we have shared with friends for nearly two decades. Now it's your turn!

2 cups desiccated coconut or coconut flakes
1 cup large medjool dates, pitted

Place the coconut in a blender or food processor and mix until the coconut becomes a little like butter.

Add the soft dates and blend until the whole mixture is soft and well combined.

Remove the mixture from the machine and spread it onto a baking tray.

If there is too much coconut oil in the mixture for your taste, 'blot' it off with kitchen paper. However, the oil is healthy and will harden in the slice.

Slice the mixture into approximately 20 squares, rectangles or triangles before refrigerating. It will be ready to eat after a couple of hours once the slice has 'set' solid. You will have to break the squares apart.

Notes

Try to use large soft dates in this recipe. If you only have small dates that are a little hard, simply heat them in a 50°C (122°F) oven for about 20 minutes until they are soft and more easily crushed. If you have a high-powered blender, then the mixture will be smoother and get warm while processing. A less powerful food processor will still produce a delicious treat.

Variation

• Use cashew nuts instead of the coconut and add ½ teaspoon ground cinnamon.

Stuffed Dried Apricots

MAKES ABOUT 10

This is an instant treat which is also nutrient dense. You can replace the hazelnut butter with macadamia, almond or cashew nut butter. Whichever nut butter you use, you will be amazed that two such simple foods can combine to produce such a luxurious and rich treat.

10 whole dried apricots
⅓–½ cup hazelnut butter

Split the dried apricots open and add 1 teaspoon of the hazelnut butter into the centre of each one.

Store the stuffed apricots in the refrigerator until ready to eat.

Variation

To turn this treat into a luxurious event, melt some dark organic chocolate (at least 70% cocoa solids or more) that contains unrefined sugar, and dip half of the apricot into the chocolate. Lay them on a silicon tray or some wax paper and refrigerate until they are set.

Note

Most dried apricots found in supermarkets are preserved with sulfur dioxide so they retain their bright orange colour. Choose dried apricots that are free from this or any other preservative. See page 66 for a list of the worst additives to avoid.

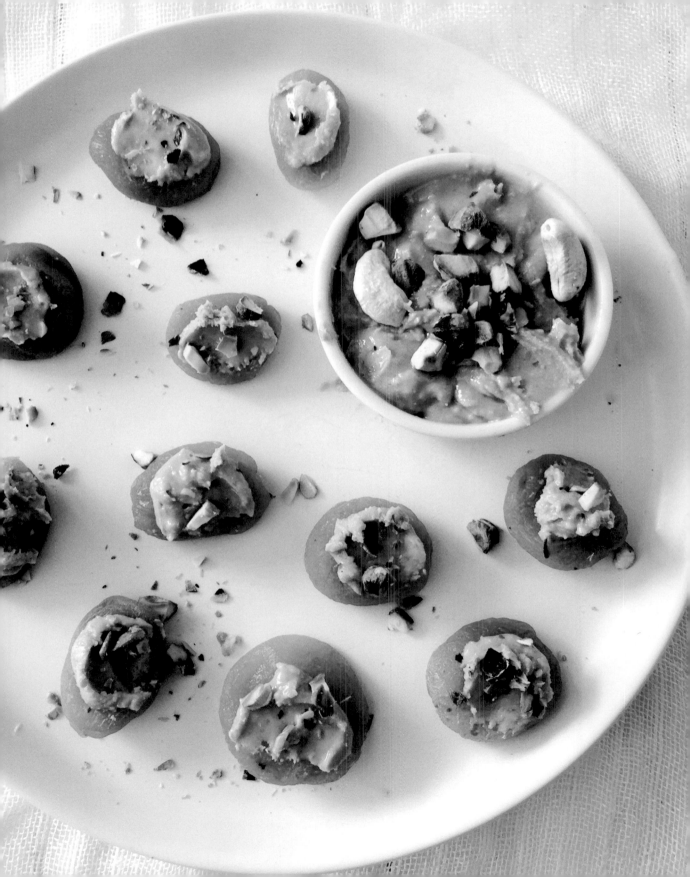

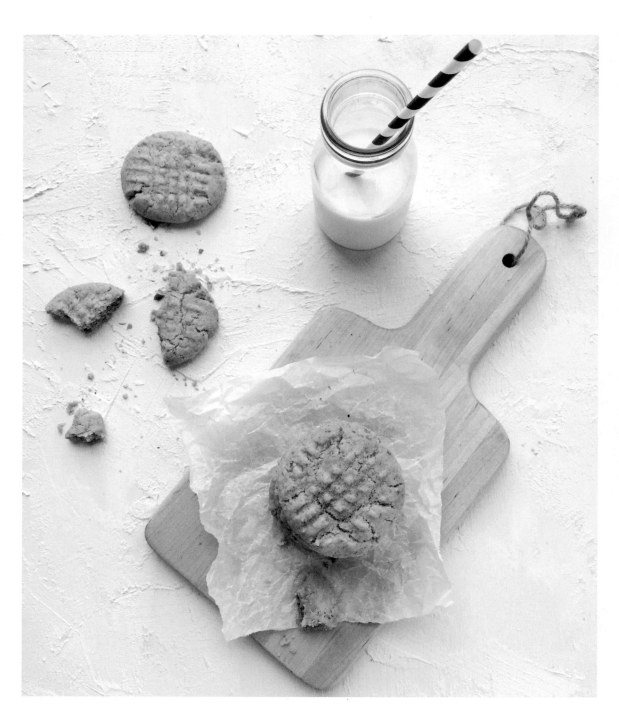

Gluten–free Vanilla Cookies

MAKES ABOUT 30 COOKIES

These delicious cookies are crispy and filling and much healthier to eat than the store-bought varieties that are full of damaging fats, sugar and gluten!

½ cup coconut or olive oil
1 cup Gluten-free Flour (see recipe on page 239)
½ cup arrowroot or tapioca flour
2 cups pecan nuts, finely chopped
½ cup unsweetened desiccated coconut
1½ teaspoons gluten-free baking powder
½ teaspoon sea salt
2 teaspoons pure vanilla extract (vanilla essence)
½ cup pure maple syrup or coconut nectar

Preheat the oven to 160°C (320°F).

Melt the coconut oil by placing it in a small saucepan over a very low heat.

In a large mixing bowl, combine the flours, pecan nuts, coconut, baking powder and salt.

Add the vanilla, maple syrup and coconut oil to the flour mixture and stir with a large spoon until a dough forms. It will be a little dry, but will quickly get softer when you roll it into balls due to the heat from your hands.

Take small pieces of the dough, roll into small bite-sized balls and place on a baking tray lined with baking paper. Press each ball with a fork to flatten them and bake in the oven for 8–10 minutes until lightly golden.

Turn off the oven, open the door and leave the cookies in the oven for about 10 minutes. Remove the cookies from the oven and leave to cool completely before storing in an airtight container.

Variations

- Add ¼ cup dark choc-chips (at least 70% cocoa solids or more) that contain unrefined sugar to the dry ingredients and toss well in the flour before adding the wet ingredients.

- Add cranberries or currants in the same way as the choc-chips above.

- Replace the pecan nuts with almonds and add 1½ teaspoons pure almond essence (almond extract) to create 'marzipan' cookies.

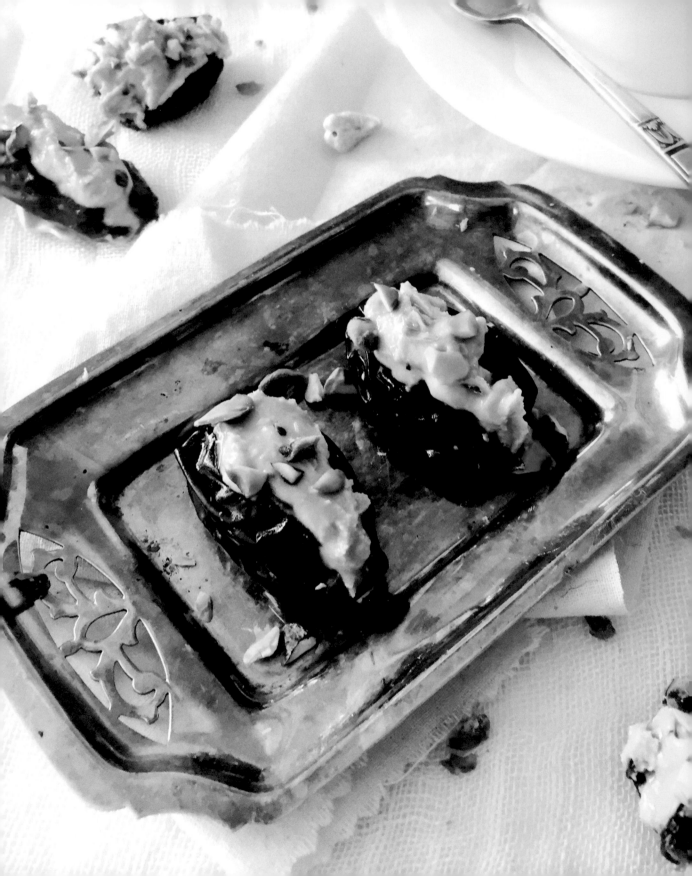

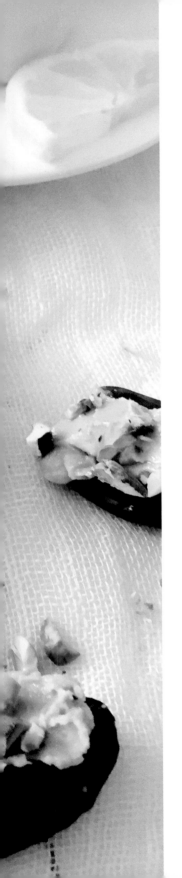

Stuffed Dates

MAKES 10

This is another instant treat! You can use any kind of nut butter such as pecan or peanut butter, but I prefer the macadamia nut butter as it is very creamy and works well with the dates.

10 large medjool dates

⅓–½ cup macadamia nut butter

Split the dates open and remove the seeds.

Insert 1 teaspoon of the nut butter into the centre of each date.

Store in the refrigerator until ready to eat.

Variation

- Melt some dark organic chocolate (at least 70% cocoa solids or more) that contains unrefined sugar, and dip half of the date into the chocolate. Lay them on a silicon tray or some wax paper and refrigerate until they are set.

Hot Chocolate

SERVES 2–3

You'll be surprised at how simple this decadent hot chocolate is to make. It's actually a meal in itself!

4 tablespoons sugar-free cocoa, raw cacao or carob powder
¼ cup cashew nuts or macadamia nuts
2 cups warmed coconut milk
3 large medjool dates, pitted
½ teaspoon pure vanilla essence (vanilla extract)
sprinkle of ground cinnamon or nutmeg, to serve
sprinkle of raw cacao nibs, for added crunch

Add the cocoa, nuts, coconut milk, dates and vanilla to a blender and mix until smooth and thick. If you have a high-speed blender, the mixture will heat up nicely if you blend it for an extra minute. Otherwise, pour the mixture into a small saucepan, place it over a low heat and stir until hot.

Pour the hot chocolate into mugs and sprinkle with cinnamon and raw cacao nibs. Serve immediately.

Variation

• If you want to transform this hot chocolate into a cold treat, simply use ice-cold coconut milk instead and replace one of the cups of water with ice cubes.

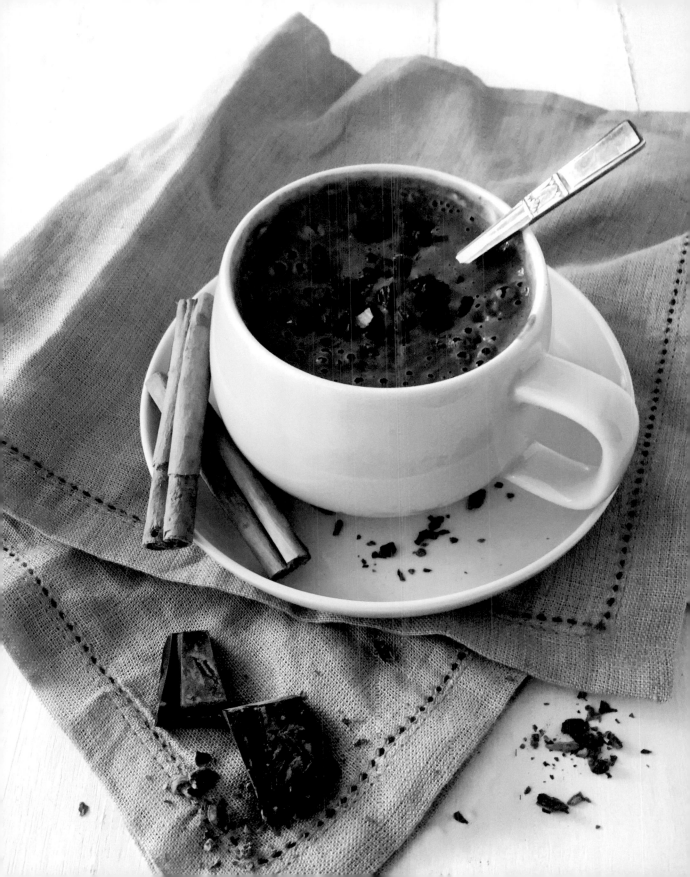

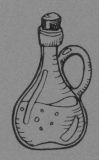

Condiments

Dips, dressings and pestos are foods that I make on the fly with whatever herbs and nuts I have on hand, but these are my staple foundation recipes. Feel free to adjust them according to whatever ingredients you have and use them in whatever way you choose. Once again you will see that these foods aim to satisfy both your taste buds and your brain, providing a range of wonderful nutrients. Adding herbs to dips, dressings or toppings adds extra nutrients to your meals with very little effort. All pestos, dips and dressings will keep in the refrigerator for up to 5 days.

Although I do not use an EFA oil blend in these recipes, I do drizzle an EFA oil on my salad after I've added my dressing of choice — the right fats keep my body and brain well-oiled and keep my skin soft and supple. I use organic, cold-pressed olive oil in my dressings and organic cold-pressed walnut, pumpkin seed (pepita), sunflower or sesame oils when I can find them.

Macadamia Mayonnaise

MAKES 1½ CUPS

Buying store-bought mayonnaise means that you are consuming a product filled with additives, flavourings and preservatives that are meant to extend the life of the product and not you! It's much healthier to make your own and you can 'tweak' it to produce endless variations! A powerful blender will give you a very smooth mayonnaise for salads, which can also be used as a spread on sandwiches or crackers with 'salady' vegetables. If you don't have a very powerful blender, then soak the macadamia nuts overnight, which will make them easier to blend together.

¾ cup macadamia nuts

juice of 1 lemon

2 tablespoons olive oil

1 teaspoon herb salt (see Notes)

cold water, as required (about ⅓ cup)

Add the macadamia nuts, lemon juice, olive oil and herb salt to a blender and combine until smooth. If the mixture gets stuck, slowly add some cold water until it starts moving again.

Store the mayonnaise in the fridge in an airtight container. This 'cream' keeps for about 5 days.

Variations

- You can substitute cashew nuts for macadamia nuts, and soaking them will make it easier to get a super creamy result.

- Add 1 teaspoon turmeric powder to the recipe just before blending together. Drizzle the resulting golden mayonnaise over salads or use as a dip for crunchy vegetables such as snap peas and asparagus.

- Add a small bunch of washed coriander (cilantro) to the mixture before blending. The resulting green mayonnaise is gorgeous as a salad dressing and can be used as a dip for roasted cauliflower (see Gluten-free and Vegan Chickpea Pancake recipe on page 217).

Notes

Some people like this mayonnaise very lemony while others prefer it less so — adjust the flavour according to your preference. This mayonnaise also makes a great 'sour cream' substitute if you add enough lemon juice to get that tangy taste. I use Herbamare® as my seasoning. It's a lovely combination of organic sea salt, herbs and vegetables, which adds saltiness to my dishes. It's available at most good health food stores and some large supermarkets.

Rosemary and Mustard Dressing

MAKES 1¾ CUPS

The Green Bean and Mushroom Salad on page 213 uses this dressing, however it is delicious with any salad, even if just sprinkled over a selection of lettuce leaves and thinly sliced red (Spanish) onion.

- 1 cup olive oil
- ⅓ cup lemon juice
- 2 teaspoons freshly chopped rosemary leaves
- 2 teaspoons dry mustard
- 3 spring onions (scallions)
- 2 cloves garlic
- 2 teaspoons maple syrup, coconut nectar or Manuka honey
- sea salt and freshly ground black pepper, to taste

Place all the ingredients in a powerful blender and blend until the rosemary leaves are finely crushed.

Store the dressing in the refrigerator in an airtight container for about 5 days.

Creamy Tahini Salad Dressing

MAKES 2 CUPS

This is a nutrient-dense salad dressing. It gets thicker as it stands and you can add some water if you find it's not of pouring consistency after a few days in the refrigerator. It's great on salads as well as a topping for baked sweet potatoes (kumera) or as a simple dip for veggie sticks.

- 1 cup tahini
- 1 cup water
- 3 tablespoons lemon juice
- 1 large clove garlic, peeled
- herb salt, to taste (see Notes on page 193)
- freshly ground black pepper, to taste
- 2 teaspoons dried Italian herbs

Place all the ingredients in a powerful blender and blend until creamy.

Store the dressing in the refrigerator in an airtight container for about 5 days.

Variations

- You can use a roasted garlic clove in place of the raw one for a richer flavour.
- I like to sprinkle some smoked paprika over the dressing before serving — it adds a rich, smoky flavour.

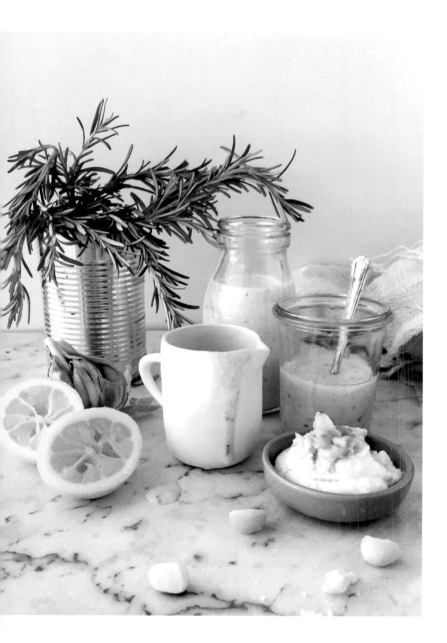

Garlic and Cumin Dressing

MAKES ½ CUP

1 clove garlic
juice of ½ lemon
¼ cup olive oil
¼ teaspoon herb salt (see Notes on page 193)
¼ teaspoon ground cumin

Blend all the ingredients together in a powerful blender. Pour the dressing over the salad of your choice and gently toss through before serving.

Variation

Add a small knob of ginger (about 1 teaspoon finely chopped fresh ginger) to the dressing mixture before blending for a more intense flavour and a little heat.

Note

Although I do use canned legumes occasionally, I prefer to use legumes that I have soaked and cooked myself. See page 242 for instructions on cooking times.

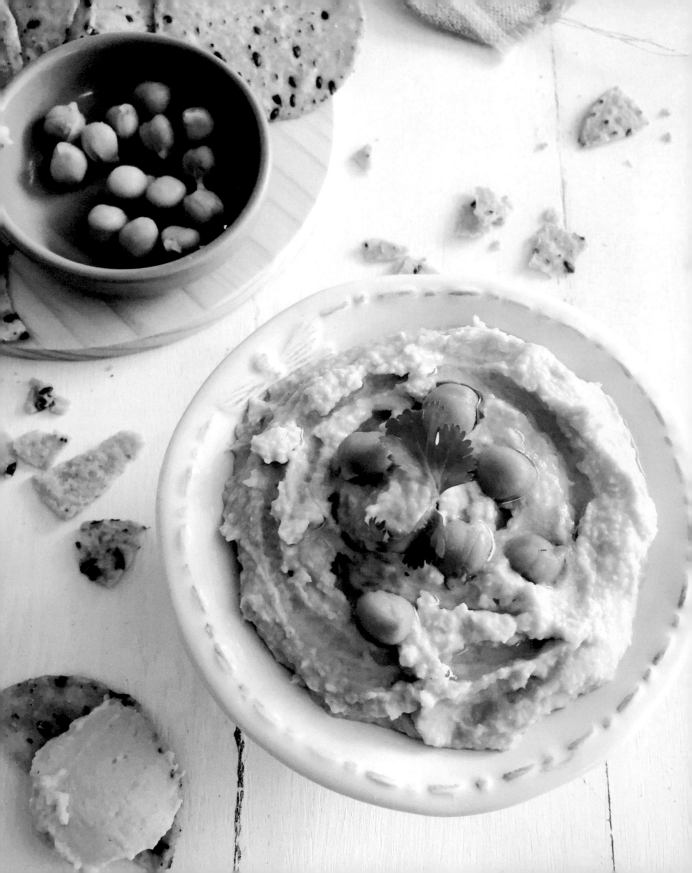

Artichoke Hummus

MAKES 1¾ CUPS

This is one of the food staples in our household. We use this dip with fresh crunchy veggies, on gluten-free bread, in baked, sweet or ordinary potatoes and on corn crackers, nachos or rice cakes. Feel free to use cannellini beans instead of chickpeas — the taste is still great! The addition of the artichokes makes it lighter, but you can leave them out and still enjoy this fabulously simple to make and nutrient-dense food!

- 1 x 425 g (15 oz) can chickpeas (garbanzo beans) or ¾ cup dried chickpeas, cooked
- 1 x 400 g (14 oz) can artichoke hearts in water
- 2 cloves garlic, peeled
- 3 tablespoons tahini
- 1 tablespoon olive oil
- juice of 1 medium lemon
- 1 teaspoon ground cumin, lightly roasted
- sea salt and freshly ground black pepper, to taste

Drain the chickpeas, reserving the liquid.

Drain the artichokes and squeeze them to get rid of the excess water inside them.

Add all ingredients, except the reserved chickpea liquid, to a food processor and blend until smooth. If the mixture is too thick, add some of the reserved liquid.

Season with salt and pepper to taste and serve.

Variations

- The addition of a roasted red capsicum (bell pepper) or even half a raw one to the basic mixture results in a delicious light 'reddish' dip. Add some finely chopped rosemary leaves to add a special flavour.

- Adding half a steamed beetroot (beet) results in a deep 'purplish' dip, and with ⅓ cup chopped mint it turns into a delicious 'twisted' version for grown-ups!

- Add a finely chopped red or green jalapeño pepper for a 'hottish' version.

- You can also add some fresh orange zest, a few tablespoons of orange juice, 1 handful of freshly chopped coriander (cilantro) leaves and ½ teaspoon of ground coriander and ground cumin for another twist.

- Instead of chickpeas use 1½ cups peas for a bright green hummus! To this you can add a small handful of finely chopped mint leaves.

Notes

I generally dribble some extra tahini over the mixture and sprinkle some ground paprika, finely chopped flat-leaf (Italian) parsley, coriander (cilantro) or garlic chives over the top. This dip is also great as part of the filling for the Chickpea Pancakes on page 217.

Onion, Garlic and Curry Jam

MAKES 1½ CUPS

4 medium onions, peeled and cut into
    eighths
6 large cloves garlic, peeled and crushed
¼–½ cup water
3 tablespoons curry powder
sea salt and freshly ground black
    pepper, to taste
2–3 tablespoons olive oil, added after
    cooking

Add all the ingredients, except the olive oil, to a
saucepan and simmer until the spices are
released. Reduce to the lowest possible heat and
allow the mixture to cook thoroughly until it
forms a 'jam'. Stir through the olive oil, turn off
the heat and use as required. You may need to
add more water if the mixture 'sticks' but the
end result should be a golden sauce or 'jam'.

Note

To make an Onion, Garlic and Italian Herb Jam
simply substitute the curry powder with 4
tablespoons dried Italian herbs. You can use this
jam on tomato-based soups and pasta. It lends a
lovely rich, mellow and buttery flavour to a dish.

Coriander Gremolata

MAKES 3–4 TABLESPOONS

This is a very fresh and vibrant
topping.

1 tablespoon olive oil
zest of 2 lemons, finely chopped
1 teaspoon crushed garlic
¼ cup chopped coriander (cilantro)

Mix all the ingredients until well combined. Use
as a topping on soups and salads or in summery
pasta dishes.

Pestos

Most pestos traditionally use cheese and mostly Parmesan cheese. Invented by the Genoese, pesto was originally made using a mortar and pestle. Today our food processors make life a lot simpler. Both of the following pestos use no cheese but are still tasty, tangy and versatile. You can substitute almonds or cashew nuts for the pine nuts. I also use walnuts, which are just as delicious! As seeds are so healthy, I've experimented with sunflower seeds and pumpkin seeds (pepitas) and have been pleasantly surprised. Pine nuts do, however, have a distinctive flavour, which is synonymous with traditional pestos.

Pestos can be used as an easy pasta sauce diluted with a little olive oil. Sandwiches are turned into gourmet treats with a spread of pesto. Pestos can be diluted with a little olive oil and lemon juice and used as salad dressings or as a tasty filling for sweet or ordinary baked potatoes. They can be used to coat roasted vegetables as they come out of the oven. Whichever way you choose to use them, pestos provide a tasty way to add valuable nutrients to your meals.

Sun-dried Tomato Pesto

MAKES 3 CUPS

It may seem like a lot of chopping needs to be done for this pesto but the end result is worth it. You can use your food processor — just blend each item individually and quickly so as not to turn everything into a soup! This mixture is good on roasted vegetables, in pasta salads and in baked sweet potatoes (kumera).

1 cup sun-dried tomatoes

1 cup pine nuts, coarsely chopped

1 cup medium-roasted red capsicum (bell pepper), finely chopped

½ cup fresh basil leaves, finely chopped

1 small bunch spring onions (scallions), finely chopped

3 tablespoons lemon juice

2 cloves garlic, crushed (use 1 clove if you don't want it too 'garlicky')

¼ cup olive oil

sea salt and freshly ground black pepper, to taste

Variations

- You can use almonds, macadamia nuts or cashew nuts in place of the pine nuts.

- If you don't have a red capsicum (bell pepper) on hand, leave it out. It doesn't affect the taste substantially.

- Replace the tomato, capsicum (bell pepper) and basil leaves with 1 cup pitted black olives and ½ cup capers to make olive pesto.

Drain the sun-dried tomatoes if in oil and soak them in water for 30 minutes until soft, then finely chop.

Combine all the ingredients in a blender or food processor until smooth. If the mixture is too stiff, add 1–2 tablespoons olive oil.

Store covered with a layer of olive oil on top in an airtight container. This pesto will keep in the refrigerator for up to 5 days.

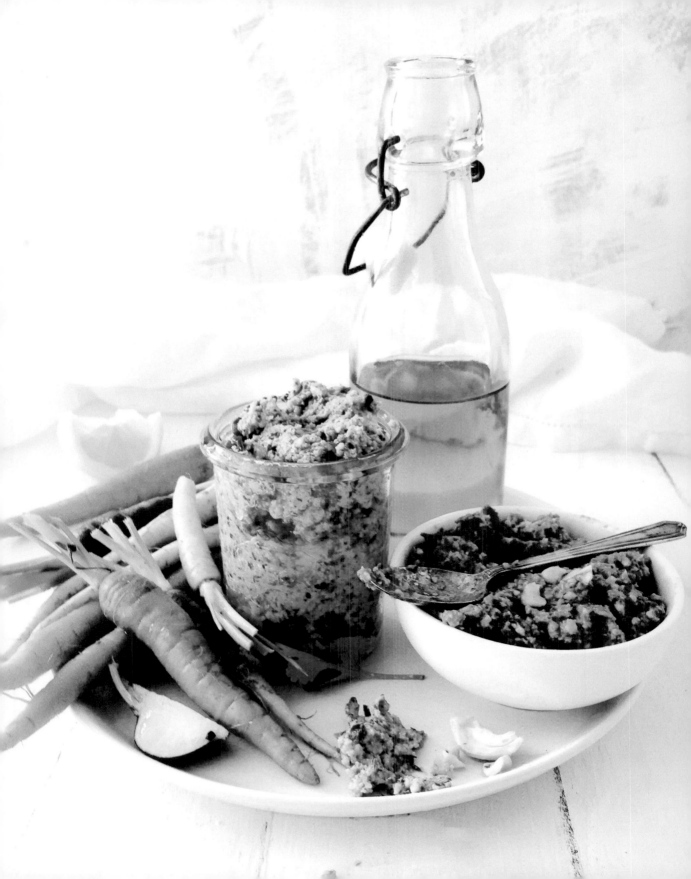

Almond Herb Pesto

MAKES 2 CUPS

We always have some form of this pesto in our fridge as it is such a tasty way to add loads of nutrients to a meal. Grow your own favourite herbs and you will be able to whip up a batch of pesto really quickly and benefit from the great green nutrients they provide.

1 small bunch chives

1 small bunch flat-leaf (Italian) parsley

1 small bunch basil

1 small bunch coriander (cilantro)

1 cup almonds

2 large cloves garlic (use 1 clove if you don't want it too 'garlicky')

2 teaspoons herb salt (see Notes on page 193)

½ cup olive oil

juice of 1 lemon

Add all the ingredients to a blender or food processor and pulse until coarsely blended. You can add a little more herb salt or lemon juice to adjust the taste. The pesto should have a herby flavour with a slight tang.

Store in an airtight container in the refrigerator for up to 5 days.

Variation

*   Replace the almonds with 1 cup desiccated coconut, the olive oil with coconut oil and use only coriander to make a delicious topping for stir-fries and vegetable soups, especially when they contain spices such as ground cumin, ground coriander or curry powder.

*   Add baby kale leaves and capers to taste to increase the nutrient content.

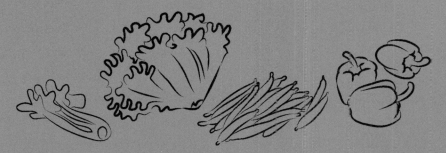

Salads and vegetables

The following recipes can easily be main meals, however you can serve them with other foods of your choice too. My aim is to introduce you to new ways of using vegetables in salads and to include them in your daily meals. Not only do green leafy vegetables contain a vast array of nutrients required by all our cells to operate optimally, they also contain fibre, which has its own special role to play in our health. I have included a list of vegetables perfect for any salad in the Basics section, so you can be creative when making salads for yourself or for family and friends. Any of the dressings and dips in this book can also be used with these salads.

I usually make enough salad in the evening to provide me with the foundation of a meal for my lunch the next day. This way I can quickly and easily prepare a midday meal. Therefore I keep my salad dressing separate from the salad until ready to eat to avoid the vegetables going limp and soggy.

I add my choice of essential fatty acids to the top of my salads and main meals, such as Udo's 3–6–9 Oil Blend, to increase the nutrient density and to provide me with these critically important compounds.

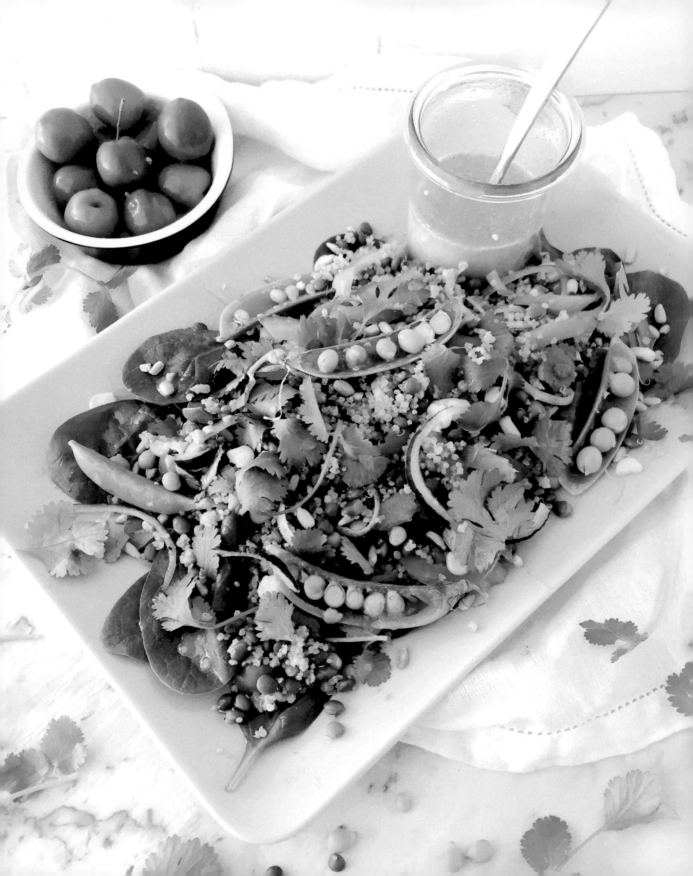

Meal-in-a-Bowl Salad

SERVES 4

This is a great salad rich in plant protein. It makes a tasty addition when served with other salads but you can serve it on its own on a bed of baby spinach leaves, rocket (arugula) or kale leaves. It also makes an excellent packed lunch the next day. You can simply eat it with a light squeeze of fresh lemon or lime juice and a dollop of olive oil as a dressing, or you can blend together the one suggested below. Either way, you'll enjoy this nutrient-dense meal-in-a-bowl.

1 cup cooked quinoa, cooled (see Basics section)

1 cup cooked lentils, cooled or 1 x 400 g (14 oz) can lentils, drained well (see Basics section)

1 cup peas (use either frozen peas which have been quickly blanched or lightly steamed fresh peas)

1 cup sweetcorn (use either frozen sweetcorn which has been quickly blanched or fresh sweetcorn which has been steamed and then cut off the cob)

¼ cup hemp seeds or sunflower seeds

2 celery sticks, finely sliced using a mandolin

1 small red (Spanish) onion, finely sliced using a mandolin

1 bunch fresh coriander (cilantro), finely chopped

½ cup green olives, pitted and thinly sliced

Simply toss all the ingredients together and serve.

You can refrigerate this salad and serve it the next day when the flavours have mingled beautifully.

Broccoli and Almond Salad

SERVES 4

The broccoli and almonds in this salad are full of easily absorbable magnesium and calcium, and paired with Creamy Tahini Salad Dressing (see page 194) it's a bone-building and calming treat! The radishes add colour and crunch. You can also add a thinly sliced red capsicum (bell pepper), for a bit of extra colour and nutrition.

1 small head broccoli, cut into florets and lightly steamed or blanched

1 bunch spring onions (scallions), thinly sliced

1 small head butter lettuce, washed and torn into pieces

1 bunch radishes, washed and sliced into strips

1 small red (Spanish) onion, thinly sliced

1 cup almonds, cut into slivers or coarsely chopped

Add all the vegetables to a large bowl and gently toss until combined.

Sprinkle the almonds over the top or serve them separately in a bowl.

Pour the tahini dressing over the salad just before serving or serve it separately as well.

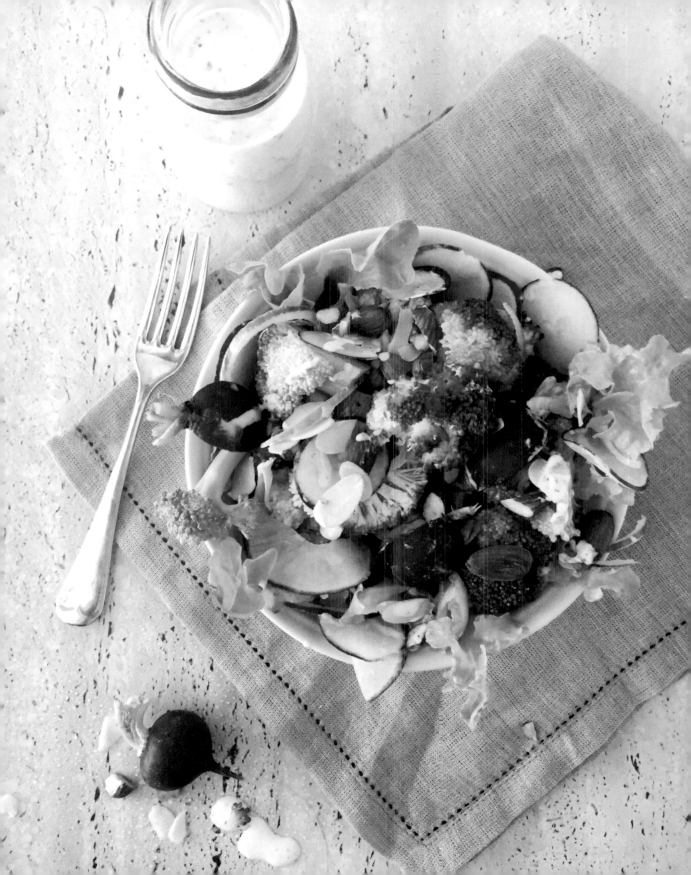

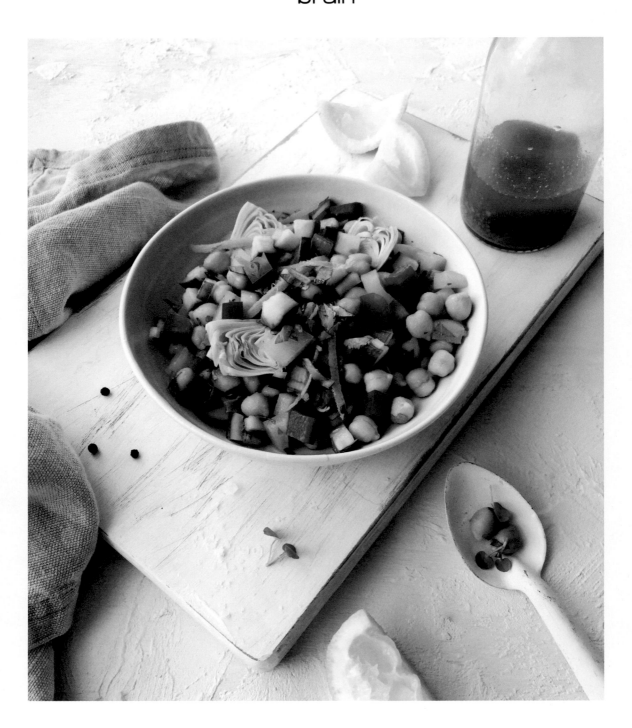

Spicy Chickpea Salad

SERVES 6

This is a substantial salad. I generally serve it with loads of fresh crispy salad leaves and ripe avocados. As a dressing, you can use the turmeric variation of the Macadamia Mayonnaise recipe (see page 193) to make it a creamy spicy salad, or just use the dressing below.

1 red (Spanish) onion, thinly sliced

1 large clove garlic, crushed

zest and juice of 1 orange

zest and juice of 1 lemon

1 large red capsicum (bell pepper), diced, or 2 roasted red peppers (bell peppers), thinly sliced

1 large yellow capsicum (bell pepper), diced

2 x 400 g (14 oz) cans chickpeas (garbanzo beans), drained

1 large English cucumber, diced

1 x 400 g (14 oz) can artichoke hearts in water, drained and thinly sliced

1 punnet (about 1 cup) fresh sprouts, washed

2–3 handfuls of rocket (arugula) or baby lettuce leaves, to serve

1 large bunch coriander (cilantro), finely chopped, to serve

Spicy Dressing

1 teaspoon ground cumin

1 teaspoon ground coriander

1 teaspoon ground turmeric

¼ cup olive oil

juice of 1 lime

To make the salad, combine all the ingredients except the coriander and rocket in a large bowl and leave at room temperature for about 1 hour to allow the flavours to develop.

Spread the rocket on a platter and spoon the salad on top.

To make the dressing, combine all the ingredients in a powerful blender.

Pour the dressing over the salad, sprinkle with the fresh coriander and serve.

Note

Use half the amount of ground cumin and ground coriander if you want a less spicy dressing.

Deli Quinoa Salad

SERVES 6–8

Quinoa is a wonderfully adaptable seed that acts like a grain, absorbing flavours very well. It is also a superb plant source of protein. This salad is a whole, satisfying meal in itself. Facing the gorgeous variety of olives, sun-dried tomatoes and artichokes at my local deli, I imagined combining a variety of those delicacies with my favourite nutrient-dense, high protein, pantry staple — quinoa. I hope you enjoy the flavour and colour of this salad. It tastes even better the next day, making it an ideal 'take-to-work' lunch.

2 cups cooked quinoa (see Note and Basics section)

1 cup artichoke hearts, drained and chopped

¾ cup olives, pitted and chopped

3 tablespoons capers, rinsed well and finely chopped

½ cup sun-dried tomatoes, finely sliced

½ medium red (Spanish) onion, finely sliced

1 cup green beans, lightly steamed

¼ cup finely chopped Italian herbs, such as basil, marjoram or flat-leaf (Italian) parsley

Dressing

¼ cup olive oil

juice of 1 lemon

½ teaspoon herb salt (see Notes on page 193)

¼ teaspoon mustard powder

1 clove garlic, crushed

1 teaspoon maple syrup, coconut nectar or Manuka honey

Place all the salad ingredients into a large bowl and gently toss until combined.

To make the dressing, place all the ingredients in a blender and blend until well combined.

This salad is best served at room temperature.

Variations

- Instead of the sun-dried tomatoes use 1 cup baby tomatoes, sliced in half.

- You can substitute the red onion with 1 small bunch of finely sliced spring onions (scallions) or ¼ cup finely sliced leeks.

Note

You need ¾ cup dried quinoa to make 2 cups of the cooked seed. Cook according to the packet instructions. You can cool the quinoa after cooking or use it warm. For this recipe, I add 1 heaped teaspoon dried Italian herbs and ½ teaspoon salt to the cooking water for extra flavour.

210

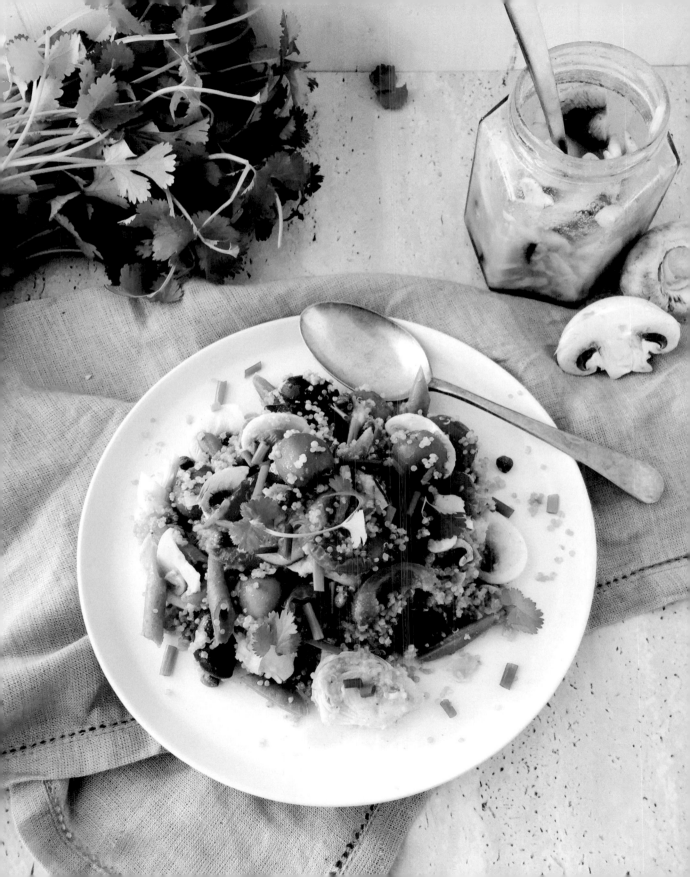

Marinated Mushrooms

MAKES 4 CUPS

This is a very simple way to maximize the unique flavour and texture of mushrooms. The great thing is that they make their own dressing while marinating, so there's no extra work when you throw a green salad together. You can easily change the kind of herbs used or add finely sliced red (Spanish) onion or spring onions (scallions) for extra flavour and colour. I love eating them with rocket (arugula) and watercress and add a few macadamias for extra crunch. However you decide to eat them, they are sure to become a staple in your kitchen.

400 g (14 oz) small button mushrooms, sliced
juice of 2 lemons
1 large clove garlic
1 teaspoon dried mustard
1 teaspoon dried Italian herbs
1 teaspoon herb salt (see Notes on page 193)
⅛ teaspoon ground nutmeg or ground turmeric
¼ cup olive oil

Put the mushrooms into a shallow glass container that has an airtight lid.

Combine all the other ingredients in a powerful blender and blend for a few seconds until well combined.

Pour the dressing over the mushrooms, stir to thoroughly coat them and leave in the refrigerator for a couple of hours or overnight, stirring regularly. The mushrooms will keep for 5 days.

Variations

- You can use these mushrooms and their dressing in an ordinary green salad.

- The mushrooms are great on steamed vegetables, baked sweet potatoes (kumera) or stirred into piping hot pasta with some chopped sun-dried tomatoes and basil pesto.

- These mushrooms are perfect with a bowl of freshly cooked quinoa.

Green Bean and Mushroom Salad with Rosemary and Mustard Dressing

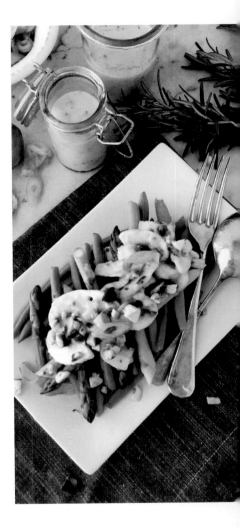

SERVES 4

This is one of the simplest salads I've ever made. The crunchiness of the mushrooms and green beans appeals to both children and adults, while the rosemary dressing is unusual and refreshing. You can use fresh asparagus when in season instead of the green beans. If you have any of this salad left over, simply refrigerate and use the next day. The vegetables will have been marinated in the salad dressing and are delicious on a bed of fresh rocket (arugula).

1 punnet (about 2 cups) button mushrooms, thickly sliced

1 punnet (about 2 cups) green beans, topped and tailed and lightly steamed

Rosemary and Mustard Dressing, to serve (see page 194)

Variation

Add crushed walnuts to increase the nutrient density.

Simply combine the mushrooms and green beans in a bowl and pour over the Rosemary and Mustard Dressing. Leave to stand for about 30 minutes before serving.

Beetroot and Pistachio Salad

SERVES 4–6 AS A SIDE

Beetroots (beets) are a generally neglected vegetable, but their nutrient content and colour are truly enticing and they are tasty too! Here's a great salad to make even though your hands will turn pink if you don't wear gloves when you 'skin' the beetroots after they've been cooked. You can eat this salad warm or refrigerate it until you're ready to serve it, although I'd let it get to room temperature first, as then the full flavour of the beetroot and herbs comes to life.

6 large beetroots (beets), leaves removed just above the stalk and cut in half

1 small bunch chives, finely chopped

1 small bunch lemon thyme, leaves removed from the woody stalk and chopped

5 or 6 spring onions (scallions), finely sliced including the green part

1 small lettuce, to serve

1 cup salted pistachio nuts, shelled and coarsely chopped, to serve

Simple Salad Dressing

zest and juice from 1 lime

¼ cup olive oil

1 small clove garlic, peeled

sea salt and freshly ground black pepper, to taste

Boil the beetroot in water for 30 minutes or until soft. They are cooked when a sharp knife slides easily into the vegetable.

Toss the herbs and spring onions in a large bowl.

When the beetroots are cooked, allow them to cool just a little, retaining some heat to release the oils in the herbs.

Cut off the beetroot tops, peel the skin and then cut them in half again so you are working with a quarter of a beetroot. Slice the quarters into slivers and toss with the herbs and spring onions. Arrange on the lettuce leaves.

To make the dressing, place all the ingredients in a blender and mix until well combined.

Pour the dressing over the salad, sprinkle with the pistachios and enjoy the gorgeous colours and flavours!

Variation

Use ½ cup freshly chopped coriander (cilantro) for a different flavour and top with walnuts instead of pistachios.

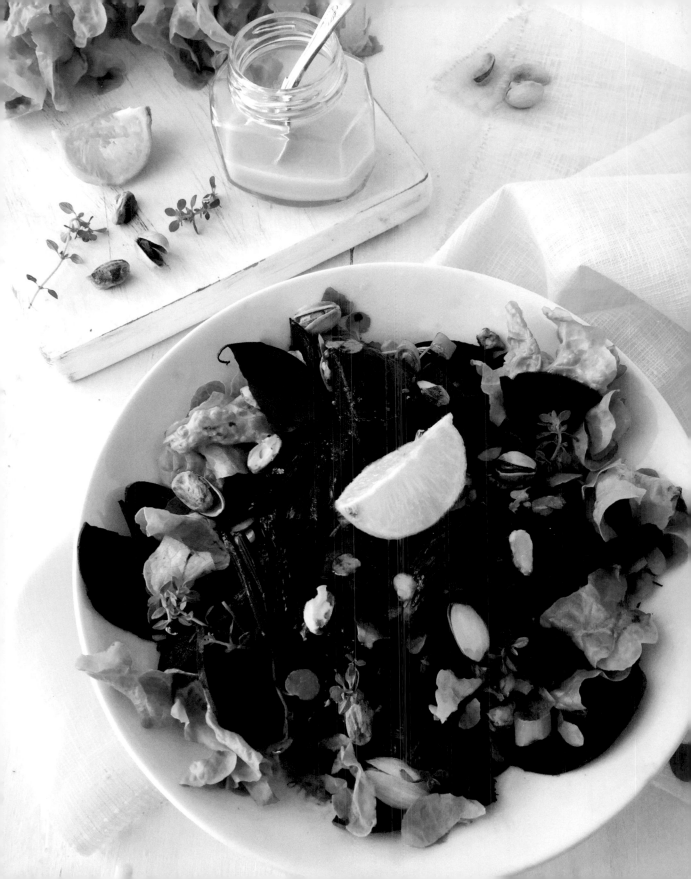

Main meals

Many of the meals in this section contain green foods either as leaves, vegetables or herbs. Eating a lot of green food provides valuable nutrients for all our cells, especially our busy brain cells! I also use legumes and quinoa and millet as they provide protein, carbohydrates and a variety of important vitamins and minerals required for optimal brain health.

You will not find any animal products in these meals. I believe that there are enough recipes available that use those foods. And although fish has traditionally been known as a brain food, our oceans are so polluted that it may not be the best choice on a regular basis anymore. Plant-based diets can provide most of the nutrients we require for optimal health and have the added advantage of not storing toxic compounds like animal products do. As you discovered in Chapter 5, it is very important to choose animal products with care if you want to nourish your brain optimally and avoid compounds that are toxic to it.

Gluten–free and Vegan Chickpea Pancake

SERVES 4

This is a very versatile recipe because you can enjoy a variety of fillings with the pancake. I make it plain and add salad, avocado, hummus, curried cauliflower, Coconut Bears (see recipe on page 220) and guacamole to make a substantial 'wrap'.

2 cups chickpea (besan/garbanzo) flour
2 cups water
¾ teaspoon gluten-free baking powder
herb salt, to taste (see Notes on page 193)
½ teaspoon ground turmeric, for colour
½ teaspoon ground cumin, to taste
1½ tablespoons lemon juice
coconut oil, as required for cooking

Add the flour, water, baking powder, herb salt, turmeric, cumin and lemon juice to a bowl and stir well until completely combined and smooth for pouring.

Melt a little coconut oil in a non-stick pan over a medium heat, then pour ⅓ cup of pancake mixture into the pan and cook while swirling the pan until you have a thin pancake. Flip the pancake and cook until the edge is lightly golden. Set the pancake aside and repeat with the remaining mixture.

Serve with the filling of your choice.

Variations

- Roasted cauliflower makes a tasty addition to pile onto these pancakes. Simply toss washed cauliflower florets in curry powder and herb salt and bake in the oven for 15 minutes at 150°C (300°F).
- Sprinkle fresh sprouts onto the pancake before rolling it up to increase nutrient density and crunch.

Note

Using ⅓ cup of the mixture makes a thin pancake, but you may need to use a little more to make a thicker pancake for wraps. It can be a bit of a messy meal but it is very tasty!

Golden Vegetable and Cashew Nut Soup

SERVES 6–8

This is a simple soup to make and the colour is simply glorious! It is a 'thickish' creamy soup, so with a large green salad and some gluten-free savoury muffins (see page 223), it makes a very satisfying meal.

1 large carrot, washed and chopped into chunks

1 medium sweet potato (kumera), washed and chopped into chunks

½ small butternut pumpkin (squash), peeled, seeds removed and chopped into chunks

1 large onion, peeled and sliced

2 cups water

1 teaspoon organic vegetable stock

sea salt and freshly ground black pepper, to taste

2 cups cashew nut milk

1 small bunch coriander (cilantro), to garnish

Add the carrot, sweet potato, pumpkin, onion, water, vegetable stock, salt and pepper to a pot, bring to the boil, then turn down the heat and simmer until all the vegetables are cooked.

Add the cashew nut milk and return to simmer then switch off the stove.

Blend the soup into a purée using a hand-held blender or simply use a potato masher.

Serve with a drizzle of cashew nut milk and a few coriander leaves.

Variations

- Use macadamia nut milk instead of cashew nut milk.

- If you want a thinner soup with a 'coconut' flavour, instead of the cashew nut milk, use 1 x 400 ml (14 fl oz) can of coconut cream with enough water to make 2 cups.

- Use the coconut and coriander pesto variation in the Almond Herb Pesto recipe on page 202 as a tasty topping.

- Use the Onion, Garlic and Curry Jam, Onion, Garlic and Italian Herb Jam or Coriander Gremolata (see page 198) as toppings to change the whole flavour of the soup.

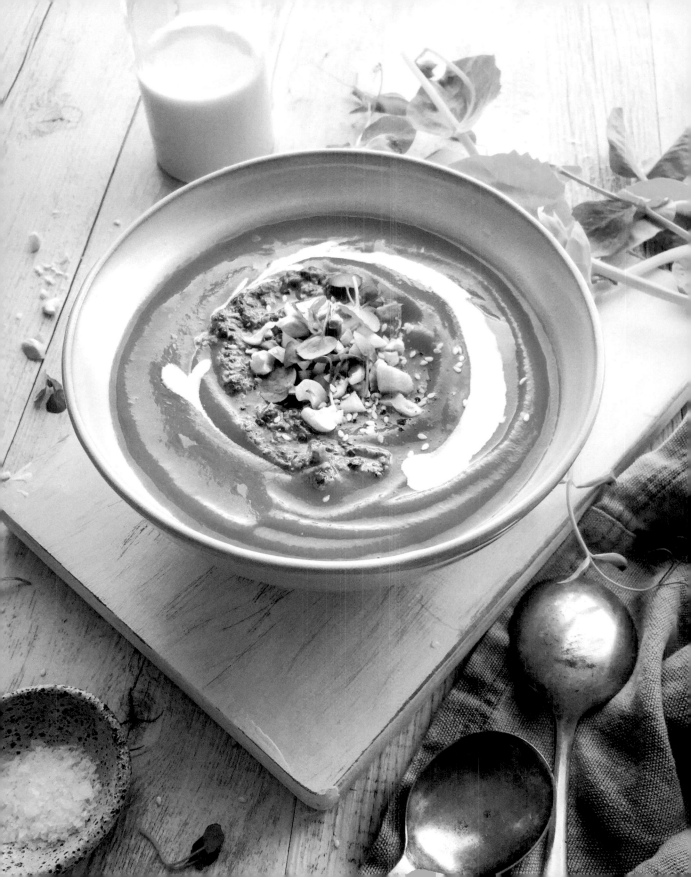

Coconut Beans

SERVES 4

This dish is the tastiest and quickest way that I've discovered to eat beans. It is a stew I serve with rice, millet or quinoa or with baked corn chips and guacamole, which is my favourite combination. It's also great with fresh corn tortillas, but rather messy! If you want to leave out the coconut cream, it's still delicious.

1 x 400 ml (14 fl oz) can coconut cream

2 teaspoons ground paprika

1 heaped teaspoon ground cumin

1 heaped teaspoon ground coriander

sea salt and freshly ground black pepper, to taste

1 medium onion, chopped

2 x 400 g (14 oz) cans kidney, cannellini or borlotti beans, drained

1 x 500 ml (17 fl oz) bottle Italian tomatoes in the form of a pasta sauce (basil and garlic or chilli work equally well)

sprinkle of finely chopped coriander (cilantro), to serve

sprinkle of finely sliced red chilli (optional), to serve

Add the coconut cream to the pot you plan to cook the stew in and place over a medium heat. Stir the cream until warm, then add the spices and onion and sauté until fragrant.

Add the beans and tomatoes, simmering until the sauce is reduced somewhat — about 30 minutes.

Sprinkle the coriander and chilli on top and serve.

Variations

- You can substitute the onion with 2 leeks or 5–6 spring onions (scallions), finely chopped.

- Add a dollop of Almond Herb Pesto (see page 202) to each serving to increase the nutrient density.

- To make a guacamole to serve with the Coconut Beans and corn chips, simply mash 3 peeled avocados with about ¼ cup finely chopped coriander (cilantro), 2–3 finely sliced spring onions (scallions) including the green part, a big squeeze of lemon juice and a sprinkle of salt.

Note

I prefer to use bottled tomatoes or tomato sauces because the lining in cans may be compromised from the acid in the tomatoes.

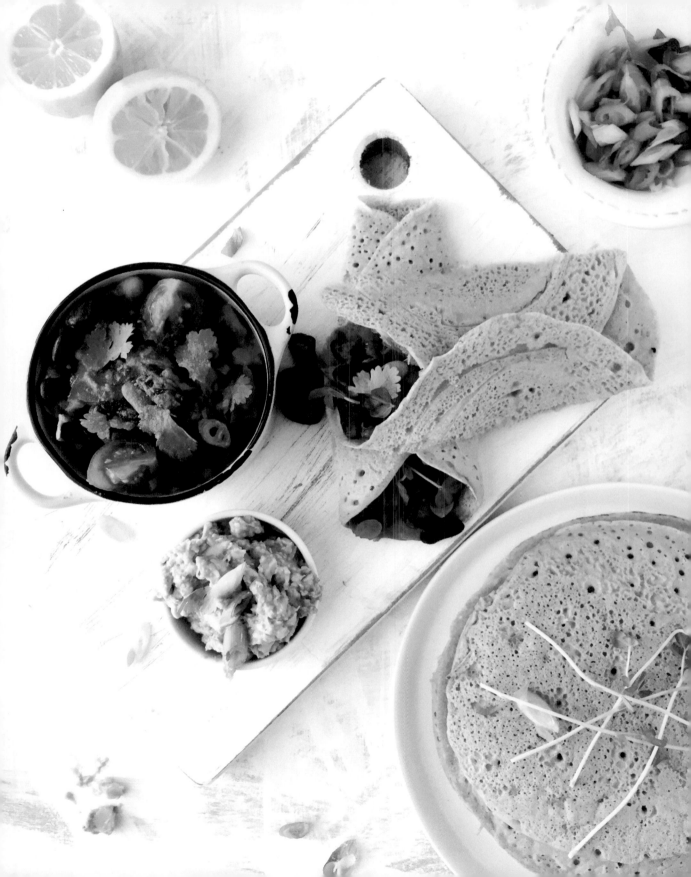

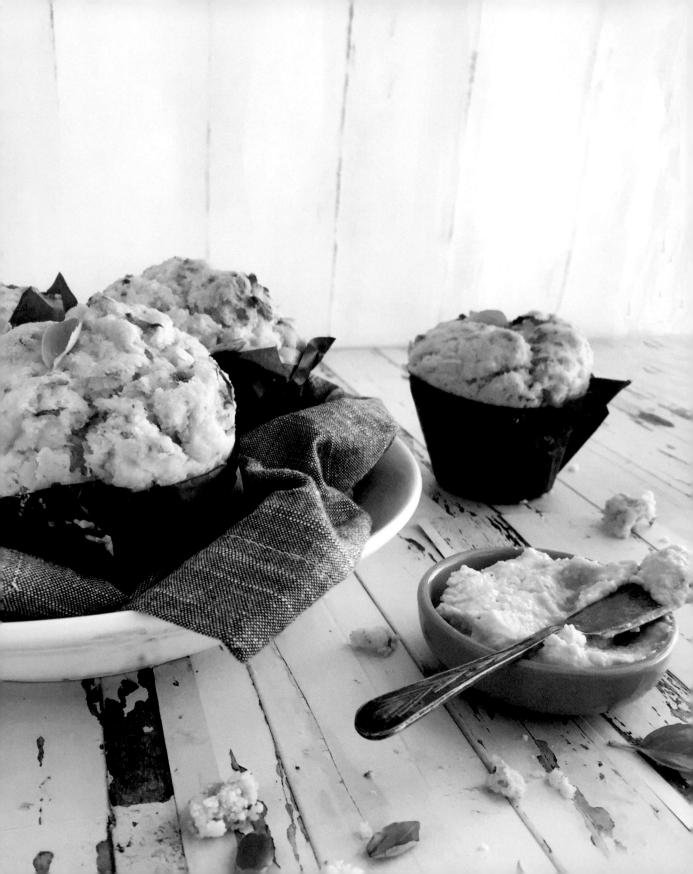

Savoury Herb Muffins

MAKES 12 MEDIUM MUFFINS

When you eat a gluten-free diet, it is not always pleasant to have to rely on rice or corn crackers or gluten-free bread. I love these savoury muffins with a piping hot bowl of soup, and they can be packed in a school lunch the next day.

1 cup gluten-free self-raising flour (see Basics section)

¾ cup almond flour

¼ cup polenta

1 tablespoon psyllium husks

1 teaspoon gluten-free baking powder

1 teaspoon dried Italian herbs

2 tablespoons fresh herbs, chopped (try a combination of flat-leaf (Italian) parsley, oregano and basil)

1 heaped cup grated carrot

¼ cup grated onion

1⅛ cups rice milk or coconut milk, at room temperature

½ cup coconut oil (see Notes)

Preheat the oven to 180°C (350°F).

Grease each hole of a 12-hole muffin tin with a few drops of coconut oil.

In a mixing bowl, combine the flours, polenta, psyllium husks, baking powder, herbs, carrot and onion. Add the milk and coconut oil and mix until well combined.

Spoon the mixture into the muffin holes until three-quarters full and bake in the oven for 20–25 minutes. Enjoy.

Variation

Add ¼ cup finely chopped sun-dried tomatoes to the final mixture for added nutrients and flavour.

Notes

You can eat these muffins for breakfast. They are delicious with mashed avocados, macadamia nut butter or hummus. If the coconut oil is solid, simply melt it in a small saucepan over a low heat until it is liquid.

Sweetcorn, Mushroom and Quinoa Pilaf

SERVES 4

One crazy weeknight I had no idea what to make for dinner and opened the fridge to find sweetcorn, mushrooms, fresh coriander (cilantro) and parsley. I decided to cook a cup of quinoa and see if these ingredients would work if thrown together. They did!

2 cups sliced mushrooms

1 medium onion, thinly sliced

2 cloves garlic, finely chopped

1 tablespoon Italian dried herbs

1 cup quinoa, cooked and cooled to room temperature

2 cups steamed sweetcorn, either off the cob or frozen

½ bunch coriander (cilantro), finely chopped

½ bunch flat-leaf (Italian) parsley, finely chopped

Place the mushrooms, onion, garlic and dried herbs into a saucepan and lightly simmer for about 15 minutes until the mushrooms dry out.

Set the mixture aside and allow it to return to room temperature.

Place the quinoa, sweetcorn, coriander, parsley and mushroom mixture in a bowl and gently toss to combine.

Serve with avocado slices and a dollop of Macadamia Sour Cream (see Note in Macadamia Mayonnaise recipe on page 193) or Almond Herb Pesto (see page 202).

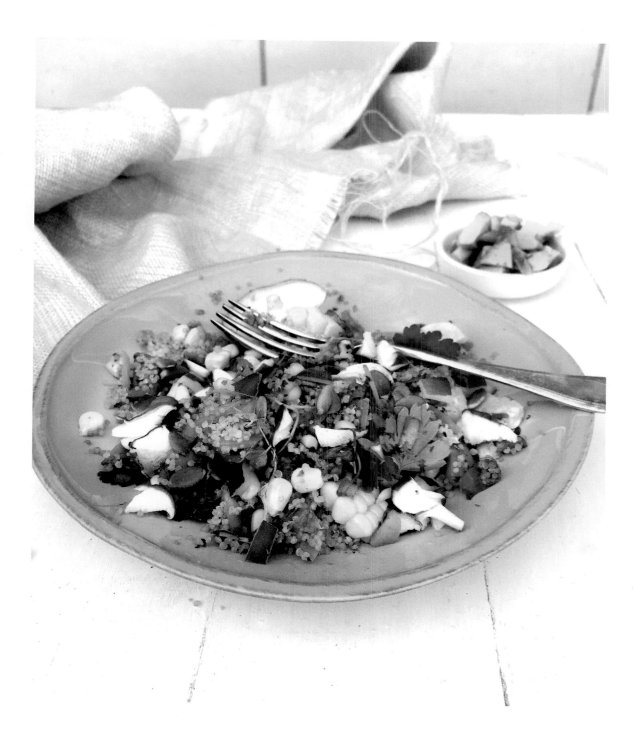

Desserts

Desserts should only be eaten occasionally due to the amount of sweetness they contain — even if it is natural and not refined! As Chapter 6 explained, our brain does not enjoy blood glucose surges, so enjoy these desserts in moderation. You will discover that my desserts are rich in nuts and oils, satisfying in mouth feel and provide valuable nutrients. In addition, you can't eat too much of them because they are super-filling! Although a number of these desserts contain chocolate, I suggest you do not consume them in the evening because the theobromine that chocolate contains can cause sleeplessness.

Raw Chocolate and Date Mousse

SERVES 6–8

Although I love using avocado in chocolate mousse, they are not always available in summer. Therefore, this recipe is my 'summer' alternative. It is very quick to make if you plan ahead and involves no cooking.

8 large medjool dates, pitted

1 cup coconut cream

1 teaspoon pure vanilla essence (vanilla extract)

1 tablespoon chia seeds

1 cup cashew nuts, soaked in water overnight

¼ teaspoon salt

6 tablespoons raw cacao powder

2 tablespoons coconut oil

fresh raspberries, to serve

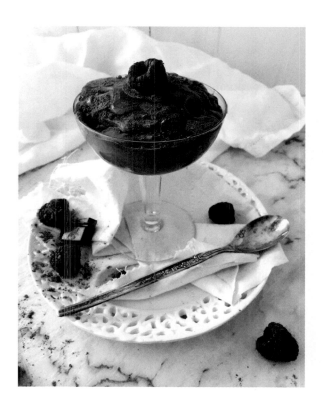

Place the dates, coconut cream, vanilla and chia seeds in a bowl and soak overnight in the refrigerator.

Rinse the soaked cashew nuts under running water until the water runs clear.

Mix the cashews, soaked dates and all the other ingredients in a high-speed blender until smooth and creamy.

Transfer the mixture to a bowl and refrigerate until firm.

Scoop the mousse into serving bowls using a warmed ice cream scoop and top with a sprinkle of cacao powder and a few raspberries.

Cashew Nut and Coconut Cheesecake

SERVES 10–12

Although this is not a true cheesecake, the texture and flavour are reminiscent of conventional 'lemony' dairy cheesecakes. It is delicious and disappears quickly when it is made.

Raspberry Topping

2½ cups frozen raspberries, thawed

2 tablespoons maple syrup or coconut nectar

Crust

2 cups coconut flakes

3–4 medjool dates, pitted

pinch of salt

½ teaspoon pure vanilla essence (vanilla extract)

Cheesecake Filling

2 cups cashew nuts, soaked overnight and rinsed well

1 cup lemon juice

1 cup coconut cream

zest of 1 large lemon

½ cup pure maple syrup or coconut nectar

1 teaspoon pure vanilla essence (vanilla extract)

¼ teaspoon salt

2 dessertspoons psyllium husks

First make the raspberry topping. Place the raspberries and maple syrup in a bowl and, using a fork, mash them together until well combined. Set aside.

To make the crust, grind the coconut, dates, salt and vanilla in a food processor until the mixture becomes soft and sticks together. The coconut will start releasing its oil and this allows the mixture to stick together when the cheesecake is put in the fridge to set.

Using a 30-cm (12-inch) pie dish, spoon the crust mixture into the dish and press it flat with your fingers to make the base. Place the crust in the freezer or fridge to set while you make the filling.

To make the filling, combine all filling ingredients in a high-powered blender until silky and smooth.

Remove the crust from the fridge and pour the filling evenly over it. Place the cheesecake in the fridge to set overnight or for a few hours at least.

Variations

- You can use blueberries instead of raspberries in the topping.

- For the crust you can halve the amount of coconut and substitute this with ground almonds or ground macadamias instead.

- Instead of the lemon zest you can use 10 drops of organic lemon essential oil in the filling.

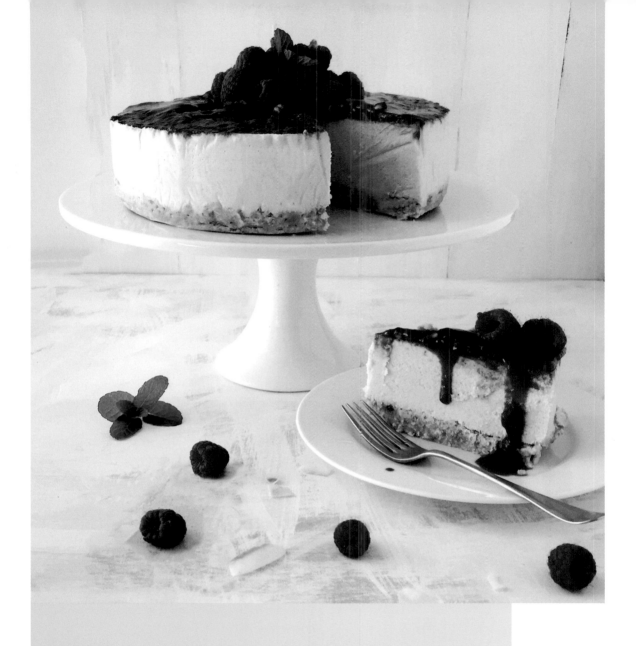

Notes

If you are in a rush you can heat the raspberries in a small pan to thaw them and then mix in the maple syrup. Allow the mixture to cool before spreading over the cheesecake, otherwise you end up with berries mixed into the cake and you lose the silky smooth centre. If you forget to soak the cashew nuts for the filling overnight, a few hours will be fine too. Using psyllium husks in the filling ensures the mixture 'sets' and has a similar texture to conventional cheesecake.

Vanilla Ice Cream with Peanut Butter Sauce

SERVES 10–12

This really is the simplest ice cream you will ever make. You can substitute the macadamia nuts for cashew nuts — the result is the same.

4 cups macadamia nuts

⅔ cup maple syrup or coconut nectar

2½ cups coconut milk

1 pinch of salt

2 tablespoons pure vanilla essence (vanilla extract)

Peanut Butter Sauce

¾ cup coconut milk

¼ cup peanut butter

⅛ cup chocolate chips (at least 70% cocoa solids or more, optional)

pinch of salt

Place the macadamias, maple syrup, coconut milk, salt and vanilla in a blender or food processor and mix until thick and smooth.

Pour the mixture into a large loaf tin, place it in the freezer and allow to freeze overnight. You need to remove the tin from the freezer about 15 minutes before serving to soften the ice cream.

To make the sauce, bring the coconut milk to a simmer and add the peanut butter. Stir until the mixture is smooth and creamy and all the peanut butter has dissolved in the milk. Add the chocolate chips and stir to combine. Stir in the salt and serve over the frozen ice cream.

Variations

- Serve with fresh cherries, raspberries and blueberries and a drizzle of coconut nectar.

- Chop up pieces of fresh mango or pineapple and stir them into the ice cream before you freeze it.

- To make strawberry or cherry ice cream, mix ½ cup fresh or frozen strawberries or cherries into the mixture, reducing the coconut milk by half. The result will be a little like a sorbet.

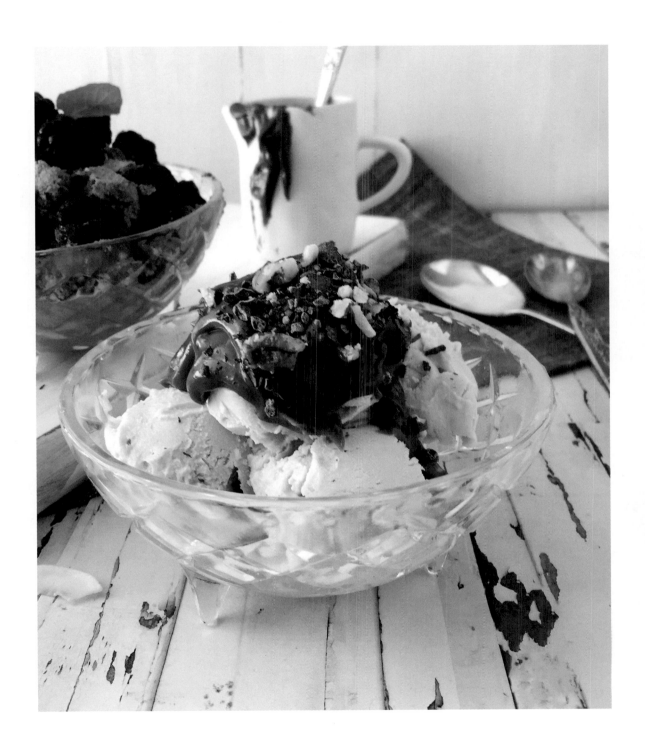

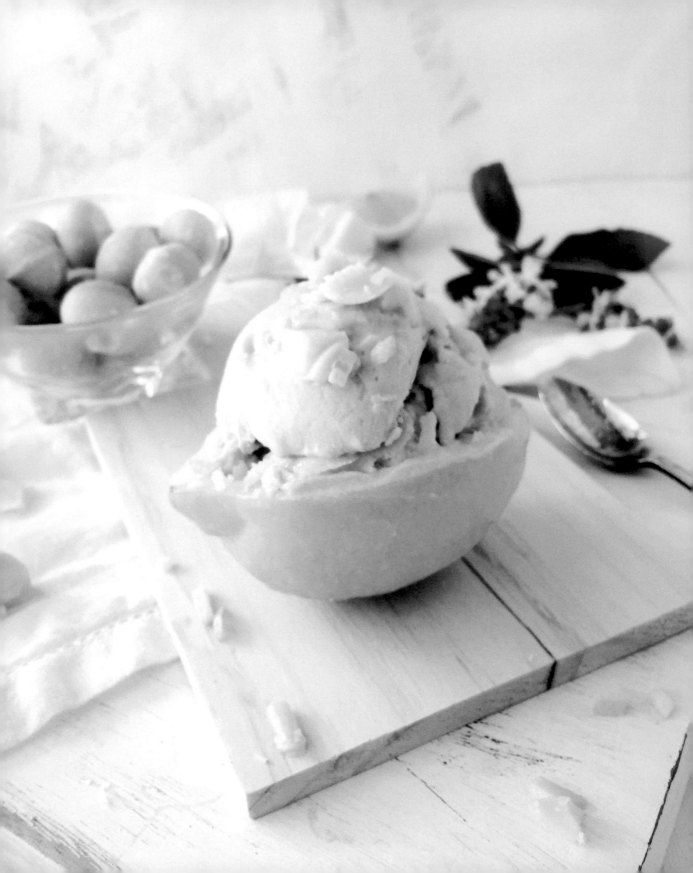

Lemon Macadamia Sorbet

SERVES 6–10

This refreshing sorbet is perfect in summer.

zest and juice of 3 lemons
1½ cups macadamia nuts
1 cup rice milk
1 cup maple syrup
5 drops organic lemon essential oil

Place all the ingredients in a blender or food processor and mix until silky and smooth.

Pour the mixture into a small loaf tin, place it in the freezer and allow to freeze overnight. You need to remove the tin from the freezer about 15 minutes before serving to soften the sorbet.

Variation

- Use the zest and juice of 2–3 oranges and organic orange essential oil in place of the lemons to make a refreshing orange sorbet.

- Serve the sorbet alone or with fresh berries or a Gluten-free Vanilla Cookie (see page 187).

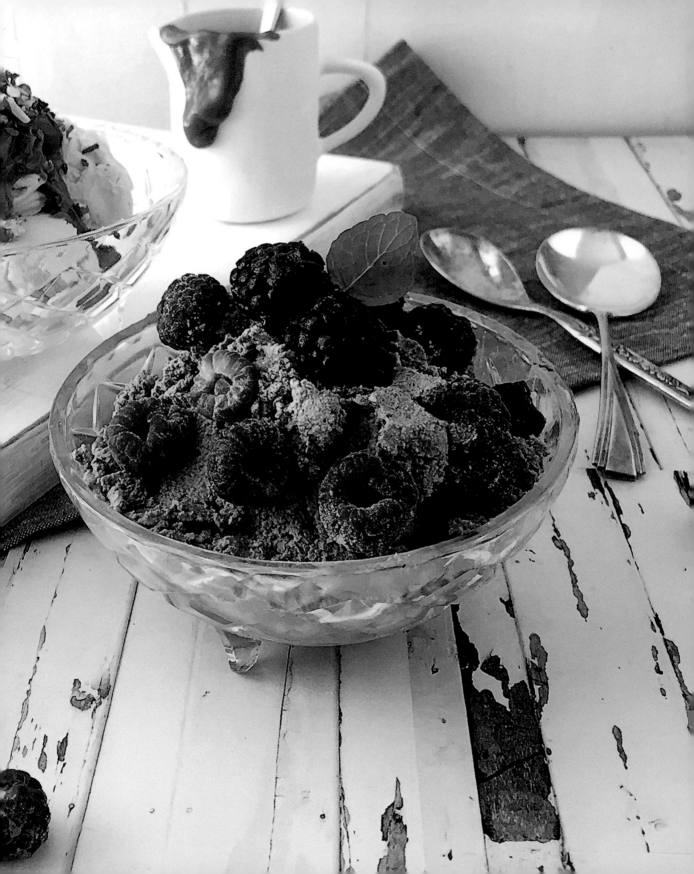

Cherry and Açai Ice Cream

SERVES 8–10

The gorgeous colours of cherries and açai as well as their nutrient status enticed me to turn them into a sweet treat using soft, sweet dates. The result is beautiful to look at and delicious, especially on a hot summer's day.

2 cup cashew nuts

1 cup cherries, pitted (see Notes)

1 cup soft medjool dates, pitted

2 teaspoons pure vanilla essence (vanilla extract)

4 tablespoons açai powder (see Notes)

1½ cups coconut cream

fresh berries, to serve

Simply combine a l the ingredients in a blender or food processor until silky and smooth.

Pour the mixture into a small loaf tin and place in the freezer overnight. Remove the ice cream from the freezer 20 minutes before serving to thaw slightly. Serve with fresh berries.

Notes

You can use frozen cherries instead of fresh ones. Açai powder can be found in any good health food store, but choose an unsweetened and freeze-dried product.

Mango Coconut Panna Cotta

SERVES 6

While enjoying a glorious mango season one year, I decided to make a simple yet elegant dessert using this golden fruit. It not only looks impressive but it tastes creamy and luscious and contains great nutrients. Be sure to use agar agar powder only, as the flakes won't work in the same way as a gelling agent.

2 cups chopped mango, plus extra pieces to garnish

2 x 400 ml (14 oz) cans coconut cream

1 teaspoon pure vanilla essence (vanilla extract)

4 tablespoons maple syrup or coconut nectar

1½ tablespoons agar agar powder (see Note)

2 tablespoons water

Purée the mango using a hand-held blender and set aside.

Add the coconut cream, vanilla and maple syrup to a small saucepan and slowly heat until everything has melted.

In a separate bowl, combine the agar agar powder and water.

Pour the agar agar mixture into the coconut cream and simmer for a few minutes stirring continuously. The aim is to dissolve all the agar agar powder, which needs heat to activate it, so that it sets when you refrigerate the dessert. Remove the pan from the heat and stir through the mango purée.

Pour equal amounts of the mixture into heatproof glasses or allow it to cool slightly before stirring and pouring into normal glasses. Allow the panna cotta to set in the refrigerator for a couple of hours and then top with the extra mango before serving.

Note

Agar agar powder can be found in any good health food store.

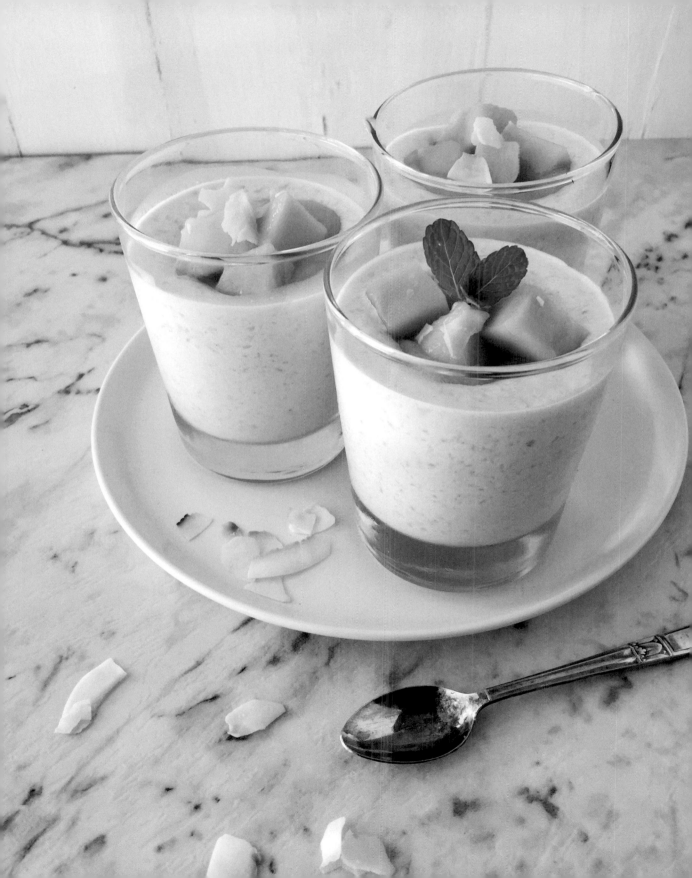

Basics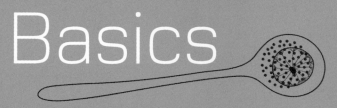

Here are a few staple recipe basics that help me 'build' other recipes. There are a few points to keep in mind:

● All the gluten-free recipes in this book use the Gluten-free Flour recipe in this section. It is rich in protein and soya free for those who need to avoid soya beans.

● The nut creams are useful in many ways, some of which I've featured in the recipes in this book.

● The vanilla essence (vanilla extract) I use is 100 per cent pure ground vanilla powder from Sunshine Vanilla (www.sunshinevanilla.com.au).

● Both quinoa and millet are great staples to have on hand. They cook quickly and easily and are perfect in a health-conscious kitchen. I have included cooking instructions in this section.

● The list of salad ingredients is a useful guide on including vegetables that aren't normally considered 'salady'. It will increase the variety and nutrient content of your salads.

● The cooking list for legumes is a guide only. Please remember to soak your legumes overnight and rinse them well before cooking.

Once you've used these instructions and recipes to prepare a variety of meals, you will find them to be staples in your kitchen too!

Nut Creams

Nuts are so versatile and can be used to make gorgeous creams for savoury or sweet dishes. Both cashew nuts and macadamia nuts can be used as a replacement for dairy cream. The only thing you need to make these creams is a very powerful blender to ensure they are smooth and creamy.

The basic ratio to make a nut cream is as follows, however the quantity does depend on how dry the nuts are:

1 cup nuts to 1½–1¾ cups water

To make a savoury cream, add 1 or 2 garlic cloves (depending on how 'garlicky' you want the cream to be), the juice of ½ to 1 lemon, some herbal salt and black pepper to the ratio above. Adjust the seasoning according to your taste.

If you are making a sweet cream, add ½ to 1 teaspoon pure vanilla essence (vanilla extract) and a pinch of salt to the ratio above. The nuts are sweet enough to not need any other sweetener, although you can add a medjool date if you need a slightly sweeter taste.

Gluten–free Flour

MAKES 4 CUPS

2 cups chickpea (besan/garbanzo) flour

1 cup brown rice flour

½ cup potato starch (see Notes)

½ cup arrowroot or tapioca starch (see Notes)

Mix all the ingredients in a bowl until thoroughly combined.

Store in an airtight container in the fridge for up to 3 months or in the freezer for up to 6 months.

Variation

If you'd like to make a gluten-free self-raising flour, simply add 1½ teaspoons gluten-free baking powder per cup of the gluten-free flour.

Notes

Potato starch and potato flour are made differently and offer different qualities to baked goods. I prefer using potato starch in this mix and suggest you do the same. Arrowroot and tapioca starch can be used interchangeably and are also sometimes called 'flours'.

Gluten-free Grains

Quinoa

Quinoa has a natural bitter coating of saponins that needs to be washed off before cooking. Some companies do this initial rinsing before packaging but others may not. It is a good idea to rinse quinoa yourself before cooking it.

To cook quinoa, use the following formula: 1 cup quinoa with 1½ to 2 cups water. It cooks in as little as 10–15 minutes. If you want it very soft, then double the amount of water, or use less for a little bite.

Place the quinoa and water in a saucepan with a lid, cover and simmer for 10 minutes. Remove the pan from the heat and allow to sit covered for 5 minutes or until all the liquid has been absorbed. Do not overcook it as it will become mushy. Quinoa is light, fluffy and translucent and triples in quantity when cooked properly. The uncooked grain should be stored in the refrigerator as it spoils quickly. Its earthy flavour is great when served hot or cold. By lightly roasting the grains before cooking, you enhance the nutty taste.

Millet

Millet is nutrient dense and a great replacement for couscous. Cooked in the way that I describe below, it is really light and fluffy.

Depending on the amount of millet you want to cook, adjust the quantities below.

Heat a medium saucepan with a lid over a medium heat and add 1 cup dry millet. Allow it to heat up then stir the grains for 3–4 minutes until fragrant. Add 2⅓ cups water and a pinch of salt and bring to the boil. Cover with the lid, reduce the heat to low and simmer for about 20 minutes after which the water should all be absorbed and the millet should be light and fluffy.

Set the pan aside with the lid still on and allow it to steam for about 10 minutes.

The Best Salad Vegetables

Use this list to create salads with ingredients you never thought of as 'salad' foods. Simply changing the way you cut a vegetable alters the way that it looks and the way you eat and enjoy it. Have fun creating new salads using the dressings I've shared with you in this book.

Artichokes: cut into pieces they elevate any salad to the sublime

Asparagus: best lightly steamed

Avocado: use liberally in any salad

Beetroot (beets): use raw, finely grated or baked in a slow oven until sweet and tasty

Broccoli: best lightly steamed and chopped into florets

Cabbage: use green, red and Chinese varieties sliced into tiny slivers

Capsicum (bell pepper): red, green and yellow varieties add colour and crunch

Carrots: sliced into circles or matchsticks they add crunch to salads

Cauliflower: best lightly steamed and chopped into florets

Celery: cut into slivers works well

Cucumber: cut into circles or matchsticks

Green beans: best lightly steamed

Herbs: use fresh in dressings or salads, including basil, flat-leaf (Italian) parsley, coriander (cilantro), rocket (arugula) and chives

Leeks: use finely chopped

Lettuce: all the varieties are perfect for salads

Mushrooms: button varieties seem to hold their shape best

Olives: always a delicious addition

Onions: use spring onions (scallions), red and brown varieties finely chopped

Peas: snow peas (mange tout), sugar snap peas and ordinary green peas in any salad

Radishes: use whole or halved for crunch, colour and bite

Spinach: best to use the small, tender leaves sliced thinly

Sprouts: a healthy and crunchy addition to any salad

Sweetcorn: best lightly steamed and off the cob

Tomatoes: the colour and taste make tomatoes a must

Watercress: a delicious, fresh addition

Zucchini (courgette): use thinly sliced or in matchsticks

Cooking legumes

Soaking legumes before cooking them removes a substance called phytic acid, which can inhibit the absorption of nutrients from the foods we eat. Soaking legumes overnight or even for 24 hours reduces the phytic acid content significantly and also helps the legumes to cook a lot faster. Be sure to rinse the legumes very well until the water runs clear before cooking them in fresh water.

Cooking times for legumes after soaking:

Adzuki beans	30–60 minutes
Black-eyed beans	1–1½ hours
Borlotti beans	1 hour
Butter beans	1–1½ hours
Cannellini beans	1 hour
Chickpeas (garbanzo beans)	1½–2 hours
Flageolets	45 minutes
Haricot beans	1–1½ hours
Lentils (large brown/green)	45 minutes
Lentils (small red)	20–30 minutes
Mung beans	40 minutes
Red kidney beans	1–1½ hours
Soya beans	3–4 hours
Split peas (large)	40–50 minutes
Split peas (small yellow)	45–60 minutes

Bring the legumes to a vigorous boil, especially red kidney beans which need to boil over a high heat for 10–15 minutes, before reducing the heat and simmering until done.

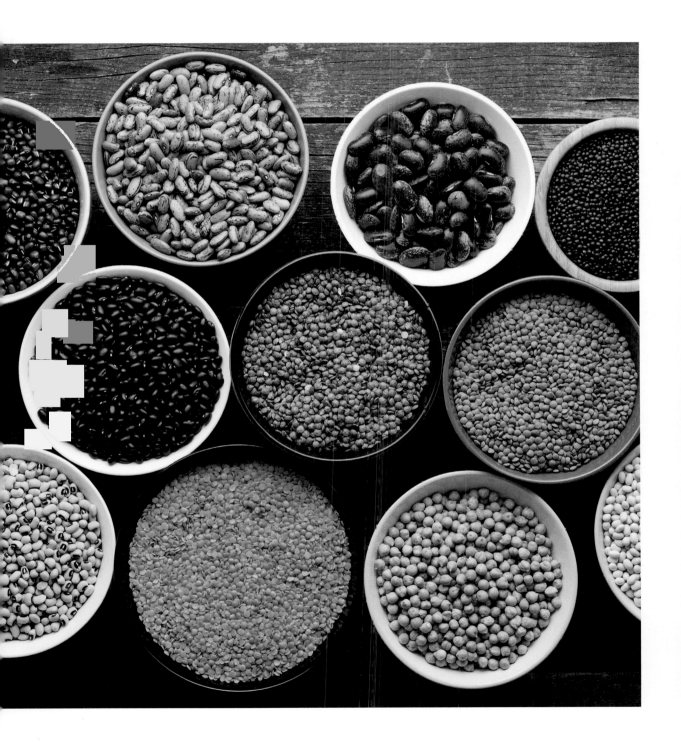

CONVERSION TABLE

Oven temperatures	
°Celsius (C)	°Fahrenheit (F)
120	250
150	300
180	355
200	400
220	450

Volume equivalents	
Metric	Imperial (approx.)
20 ml	½ fl oz
60 ml	2 fl oz
80 ml	3 fl oz
125 ml	4½ fl oz
160 ml	5½ fl oz
180 ml	6 fl oz
250 ml	9 fl oz
375 ml	13 fl oz
500 ml	18 fl oz
750 ml	1½ pints
1 litre	1¾ pints

Weight equivalents	
Metric	Imperial (approx.)
10 g	⅓ oz
50 g	2 oz
80 g	3 oz
100 g	3½ oz
150 g	5 oz
175 g	6 oz
250 g	9 oz
375 g	13 oz
500 g	1 lb
750 g	1⅔ lb
1 kg	2 lb

Cup and spoon conversions

1 teaspoon = 5 ml

1 tablespoon = 20 ml

¼ cup = 60 ml

⅓ cup = 80 ml

½ cup = 125 ml

⅔ cup = 160 ml

¾ cup = 180 ml

1 cup = 250 ml

Glossary

Adenosine triphosphate (ATP)

ATP is called the universal molecule of energy and is produced in the mitochondria of cells via the breakdown of carbohydrates or other foods. It is the form of energy that all cells use to perform the functions that keep us alive.

Adrenaline

Adrenaline is secreted by the adrenal glands when the brain perceives a stressful event or thought. Blood circulation, rate of breathing and carbohydrate metabolism increase, all in anticipation of either flight from or fight with the perceived danger. Adrenaline is also known as epinephrine.

Advanced glycation end products (AGEs)

AGEs are compounds formed when heat and oxygen change the composition of sugar or protein molecules in food, or when we consume sugars that interact with the proteins in our body. AGEs are extremely damaging and can lead to several lifestyle-related diseases, inflammatory conditions and brain ageing.

Alpha-linolenic acid (ALA)

A short-chain omega-3 fatty acid.

Amines

Amines are compounds that are formed by the breakdown of proteins in specific foods. Some hormones also contain amines, such as adrenaline (epinephrine), serotonin and dopamine. If you are taking a monoamine oxidase inhibitor (MAOI), you will need to avoid consuming foods that contain amines.

Amygdala

The amygdala is an almond-shaped mass of grey matter that is part of the limbic system in the brain. It has numerous extensions to the olfactory (nasal) system and sends nerve fibres to the hypothalamus. Its functions are related to the perception of threat, fear, emotion, learning and memory.

Anaemia

Anaemia is a condition in which the blood does not contain enough red blood cells or haemoglobin. Anaemia is very serious for the brain because without the oxygen and nutrients carried by the blood, the brain cannot function optimally. There is also an increased risk of dementia in the presence of anaemia.

Anthocyanins

Anthocyanins are water-soluble compounds that provide purple, blue and red colouring to plants and flowers. They are potent anti-oxidants.

Anti-oxidant

Our cells use glucose and oxygen to make energy. Free radicals are produced during this process. Free radicals are unstable compounds and by donating an oxygen molecule, anti-oxidants stabilize them, thereby stopping them from damaging healthy cells. The brain produces enormous quantities of free radicals and anti-oxidants can help protect neurons from free radical damage. Common examples of potent anti-oxidants are vitamin C, vitamin E and beta-carotene, the precursor to vitamin A.

Arachidonic fatty acid (AA)

An arachidonic fat molecule is an omega-6 polyunsaturated fatty acid. It has eighteen carbon atoms in its molecular chain and four double bonds. It is found in animal products and can be synthesized from some plant forms of omega-6. It is often described as being a 'bad' fat but it has critically important roles to play in the brain.

Aspartame

Aspartame is an artificial sweetener made up of three different substances: aspartic acid, phenylalanine and methanol (wood alcohol). These substances are released into the bloodstream when ingested and have been linked to numerous health challenges, including cognitive problems.

Aspartate

Aspartate is an amino acid used in the brain as a neurotransmitter. It is considered to be an excitotoxin when consumed in high doses, causing damage and even death to sensitive neurons. It is found in some artificial sweeteners, such as aspartame.

Axon

An axon is the extension of a neuron that carries information away from the neuron to neighboring cells via their dendrites. The communication from axon to dendrite occurs at the site of a synaptic junction, where neurotransmitters 'jump' across the gap sending messages in a continuous stream.

Benzoates (benzoic acid)

This compound is found naturally in some foods, however sodium benzoate is produced commercially and is used a preservative in processed foods.

Beta-amyloid

Beta-amyloid is a protein that circulates in human blood and cerebrospinal fluid (CSF) and which can be deposited into plaques (a sticky substance that clings to neurons) in the brains of Alzheimer's sufferers. It is also called amyloid-beta protein.

Glossary

Bio-identical hormone replacement therapy (BHRT)

BHRT is a form of complementary medicine where hormones which have the same chemical formula as those made naturally in the human body are used to help balance hormone fluctuations and to restore normal levels. It can be used by both men and women.

Blood–brain barrier

The blood–brain barrier is a specialized system of cells that form a barrier against certain harmful compounds entering the brain. These specialized cells can be compromised in their protective function during certain infectious states, after head injury and in degenerative conditions. Some parts of the brain never develop a barrier at all, so it is not a perfect solution against neuronal toxic uptake. The barrier is also not fully functional in youth and old age.

Brain-derived neurotrophic factor (BDNF)

BDNF is a specific protein that encourages neuronal health and dendrite production, as well as helping to spur on the growth of new neurons (neurogenesis). It is intricately involved with brain plasticity, allowing the brain to change and grow depending on the circumstances and situations it finds itself exposed to.

Casomorphin

During the process of digestion, specific proteins are broken down into opioid-like compounds which are thought to act on the opioid receptor sites in the brain eliciting feelings of pleasure and enjoyment. Casomorphin is a compound found in dairy products thought to elicit this kind of response.

Central nervous system (CNS)

The CNS is a sophisticated and complex group of nerve tissues that control all the activities of the body. It is made up of the spinal cord and the brain. It is responsible for co-ordinating and controlling all the nervous activities that arise from both internal and external mental and physical stimulation.

Cerebrospinal fluid (CSF)

Cerebrospinal fluid is a clear, watery fluid that surrounds the brain and spinal cord. It is made up of white blood cells, glucose, salts and enzymes.

Cholesterol

Although cholesterol is classified as a fat or lipid, it is actually a steroid which is part of a group of compounds that are responsible for synthesizing hormones and regulating inflammation among other things. The balance of cholesterol is critically important for optimal cell membrane functioning. Low-density lipoproteins (LDLs) and high-density lipoproteins (HDLs) are tiny compounds that help to carry cholesterol from the liver to various tissues and cells in the body.

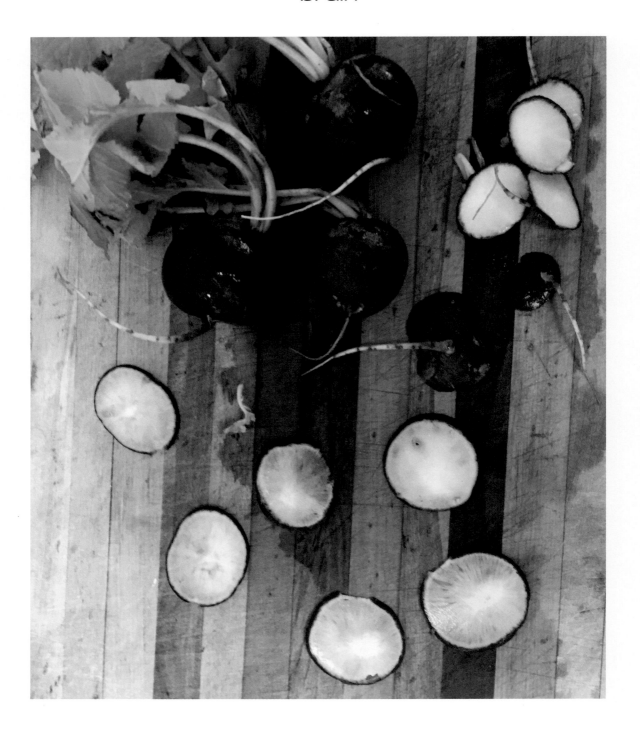

Glossary

Choline

Choline is a compound that is found widely in living tissues and is capable of being produced in the liver. It is involved in the transport of lipids (fatty acids) in the body. It is found in lecithin, as well as in eggs and other proteins. Choline is the precursor to the neurotransmitter acetylcholine.

Cortisol

Cortisol is a hormone that is produced by the adrenal glands and required for normal endocrine function. It is produced in response to long-term stress. It influences the metabolism of fats, carbohydrates and proteins, and when produced in excess causes inflammation among other things. It is also involved in the immune system and blood pressure regulation.

Cysteine

Cysteine is an amino acid found in the protein keratin, which is present in skin, hair and nails. It is also found in many enzymes.

Dendrite

Dendrites are the tiny, branched extensions of the neuron that collect electrochemical signals from other neurons to pass on to the cell body they are attached to. Their branched characteristic allows them to have a large surface area from which to receive many signals from many axons, allowing the signals to flow simultaneously to many different target neurons.

Deoxyribonucleic acid (DNA)

DNA is the genetic material of living things which controls what is inherited from predecessors. It is found in the cell's nucleus on structures called chromosomes. DNA makes exact copies of itself, passing on information to the cells when the cell divides. Changes in the DNA cause mutations to the cells.

Docosahexaenoic acid (DHA)

A DHA fat molecule is an omega-3 fatty acid that has six double bonds and 22 carbon atoms in its molecular chain. It is the most sophisticated and chemically active fat molecule known. It is found in large quantities in the brain.

Eicosanoid

An eicosanoid is a special substance that acts like a hormone, in that it passes messages between cells. Eicosanoids act locally and on specific cells close to where they are formed. All the eicosanoids have twenty carbon atoms in their molecular structure with differing double bonds, just like the essential fatty acids they are derived from. They have complex acronyms according to their specific molecular structure and how many double bonds they have. They are involved in a huge number of regulatory functions throughout the body, including the central nervous system (CNS). They regulate inflammation, blood pressure, immune functioning, reproductive processes and tissue growth, among other functions. The various networks of cells, tissues and organs that depend on the eicosanoids for optimal functioning are some of the most complex in the human body. They largely explain the phenomenal health benefits of consuming omega-3 and omega-6 fatty acids.

Eicosapentaenoic acid (EPA)

An EPA fat molecule is an omega-3 fatty acid that has five double bonds and twenty carbon atoms in its molecular chain. It is the second-most sophisticated and chemically active fat molecule known. It is found in large quantities in the brain.

Endorphins

Endorphins are a group of hormones that are produced within the central nervous system (CNS). They have a number of different functions, one of which is to activate the body's opiate receptors, which leads to a reduction in pain.

Essential fatty acids (EFAs)

These fats are 'essential' because the body cannot make them. They have to be supplied by your diet. Both omega-3 and omega-6 are EFAs.

Estrogen (Oestrogen)

Estrogen is one of a group of hormones that regulate female sexual development and the functioning of female sexual organs, as well as secondary sexual characteristics such as breasts. Estrogen is produced in the ovaries and in smaller amounts in the adrenal glands. Both natural and synthetic forms of estrogen are used to balance hormonal fluctuations. Synthetic, or what are called environmental estrogens, are also found in meat, milk plastics and pesticides, leading to an over-supply of estrogen in human cells and tissues.

Excitotoxin

Excitotoxins are a group of excitatory neurotransmitters that can cause the death of sensitive neurons. Some of these compounds are found in foods, such as tomatoes and mushrooms, and are harmless if eaten in moderation. Aspartate is known to be an excitotoxin when consumed at high doses, such as in some artificial sweeteners.

Exorphins

Exorphins have a similar action to endorphins, but they originate outside the body. An example is morphine. They are made up of tiny proteins called peptides, which both gluten and dairy contain in small quantities.

Fatty acids (FAs)

A fatty acid (FA) is a fat molecule that has a fatty end, which is water insoluble and an acid end, which is water soluble. This simply means the fatty end repels water and dissolves in oil, while the acid end dissolves in water. This is why they work so well in cell membranes. Fatty acids can vary in length. Different numbers are assigned to them, depending on how long their chains are.

Free radicals

Free radicals are highly reactive compounds that are formed during the production of energy using oxygen within cells. They can cause damage to cell components, including the mitochondria, leading to further free radical production. Anti-oxidants counter the damage that free radicals cause, donating electrons to these unstable compounds to make them stable again.

Gamma-aminobutyric acid (GABA)

GABA is an inhibitory neurotransmitter. It reduces activity in neurons, helping to maintain balance and equilibrium in the brain between neuronal activity and rest. It may reduce the states of anxiety and fear in the brain.

Gamma-linolenic fatty acid (GLA)

This is an omega-6 polyunsaturated fatty acid. It is made up of eighteen carbon atoms in its molecular chain and has three double bonds. It is made in the human body from plant forms of omega-6 or obtained directly from other plants, such as evening primrose oil.

Ghrelin

Ghrelin is an enzyme produced by cells in the stomach lining which stimulate appetite. Ghrelin works with both leptin and insulin to monitor food intake and satiation.

Glucose tolerance factor (GTF)

GTF is a water-soluble compound containing both chromium and nicotinate, which help to regulate blood glucose tolerance. It influences insulin function as well. When GTF is not functioning optimally, along with a number of other factors, glucose intolerance occurs. It is a term used to signify a number of metabolic conditions where higher than normal blood glucose levels are observed. Lifestyle choices are leading to increased cases of glucose intolerance, such as Type 2 diabetes, pre-diabetes, metabolic syndrome, impaired glucose fasting and impaired glucose tolerance.

Glutamate

Glutamate is an excitatory amino acid that is used by the brain as a neurotransmitter. In high concentrations it becomes toxic to neurons becoming an excitotoxin.

Glutathione

Glutathione is a potent anti-oxidant that the body produces and which protects against free radical damage. It is also important in ensuring optimal function of proteins, membrane lipids (fatty acids) and haemoglobin. High levels in the blood are associated with longevity. It can be taken in supplement form.

feed
your
brain

Gluteomorphin

During the process of digestion, specific proteins are broken down into opioid-like compounds, which are thought to act on opioid receptor sites in the brain, eliciting feelings of pleasure and enjoyment. Gluteomorphin, a compound found in gluten-containing grains, is thought to elicit these responses. It is also known as gliadorphin, another protein found in gluten-containing grains.

Glycine

Glycine is an amino acid found in most proteins. It also functions as an inhibitory neurotransmitter.

Glymphatic system

The glymphatic system is a 'process' by which cerebrospinal fluid (CSF) moves through channels in the brain cleansing it of toxic debris, particularly during sleep. It is also known as a functional waste-clearing pathway for our central nervous system (CNS).

Hippocampus

The hippocampus is a region of the brain located in the temporal lobe. It appears to play a significant role in memory, as well as learning and emotion, connecting them in ways that allows long-term memory consolidation and retrieval to function effectively. It is a source of neural stem cells, which makes it a very important part of the brain. It is damaged by ongoing stress.

Histamine

When cells are injured, or when they respond to an allergy-causing substance such as pollen, they release histamine which causes a dilation of blood capillaries and the contraction of smooth muscle fibres. A runny nose and sneezing are two of the most common reactions that histamine-containing cells produce. If you are taking a monoamine oxidase inhibitor (MAOI), you will need to avoid consuming foods that contain histamine.

Homocysteine

An amino acid that occurs as an intermediate step in the metabolism of cysteine and methionine. Elevated levels of homocysteine in the blood have been linked to an increased risk of cardiovascular disease (CVD).

Hormones

A hormone is a chemical compound that is produced in the body often by special glands such as the thyroid or ovaries. Hormones regulate or control the activity of specific cells, tissues or organs. They can also be thought of as special messengers, constantly regulating and keeping various systems working in balance. They are involved with growth and development, reproduction and metabolism. As we age, their synthesis can become less reliable.

Hypothalamus

The hypothalamus is a region of the brain below the thalamus that co-ordinates or manages the autonomic nervous system, the pituitary gland, body temperature, hunger, thirst, sleep, sex and emotions. It also regulates the release of specific hormones. If it isn't working efficiently, the entire body and brain will be in a state of disequilibrium.

Hypothalamus-pituitary-adrenal axis (HPA axis)

The HPA axis is a complex and sophisticated set of instructions and feedback loops that occur between the hypothalamus, the pituitary gland and the adrenal glands. These endocrine glands are involved in the activation of the stress response and work together to provide feedback to each other, which can minimize the damage that the ongoing production of cortisol can lead to.

Immunoglobulins

Antibodies known as immunoglobulins are produced by the immune system in response to being exposed to a possible allergen. The body produces various kinds of antibodies including immunoglobulin E (IgE), and immunoglobulin G (IgG). IgGs are the most prolific antibodies in the body and fight viral and bacterial infections, and may be useful in detecting food intolerances. IgEs bind to allergens and trigger the release of mast cells leading to inflammation.

Insulin

Insulin is a hormone which regulates the amount of glucose that is circulating in the blood. Insulin promotes the use of glucose for energy by cells, and anything that interferes with either its production or its availability to cells will lead to blood glucose fluctuations and eventually diabetes.

Leptin

Leptin is a hormone produced by fat cells which regulates fat storage in the body. The hypothalamus contains leptin receptors which instigate the satiation response when enough food has been consumed to satisfy appetite. It is also involved with metabolism and works with insulin and ghrelin to keep blood glucose and weight stable.

Linoleic acid (LA)

An omega-6 fatty acid.

Lymphatic system

The lymphatic system is a network of organs, nodes, ducts and vessels which move fluid from tissues into the bloodstream.

Melatonin

Melatonin is a sleep-specific hormone that is produced in the pineal gland from the neurotransmitter serotonin when a lack of light is perceived via the eyes, indicating that night is approaching and sleep is imminent. It is intricately related to our sleep and wake cycles.

Methionine

Methionine is an essential amino acid found

in most proteins. It is involved in an intricate process called methylation, which keeps neurotransmitters, hormones and other important chemicals in balance. SAMe is also involved in this process.

Methylsulfonylmethane (MSM)

MSM is a sulfur-containing compound found naturally in many foods. Due to its sulfur content it is often used as part of a detoxification program. It is also used as a natural remedy for joint pain and may be a general anti-inflammatory. It plays a vital role in the production of glutathione, an important anti-oxidant.

Mitochondria

These are tiny factories that produce energy within our cells. Adenosine triphosphate is one of the types of energy it produces, mainly from the carbohydrates we consume combined with oxygen. Mitochondria move around the neuron, axon and dendrite, meeting demands for its energy supply as needed. Exercise can increase their number.

Monosodium glutamate (MSG)

MSG is the sodium salt of glutamate and has the same excitotoxin properties of pure glutamate. It has been linked to many physical and mental challenges, from digestive upsets to seizures.

Monounsaturated fatty acids (MUFAs)

A monounsaturated fatty acid (MUFA) is a fat molecule that has one double bond in its molecular chain. Monounsaturated fatty acids (MUFAs) can have anywhere from ten to eighteen carbon atoms in their chain, but the most important one has eighteen and its double bond between carbons eight and nine. It is called 'oleic' acid and is the predominant type of fat found in olive oil. Olive oil is also an omega-9 because it has one double bond between carbon atoms nine and ten. The body can make omega-9 monounsaturated fatty acids (MUFAs).

Myelin

Myelin is a specialized, fatty, sheath-like form of insulation that covers the axon of a neuron. Myelin helps the electrical impulse that travels along the axon to the next nerve cell to move at very high speeds. When myelin gets damaged, the communication between neurons is severely hampered. The composition of myelin is largely dependent on the types of fats and oils we eat. Myelination is the process by which the fatty layer or sheath accumulates around the axon.

Neurochemical

A neurochemical is a molecule, such as a neurotransmitter (serotonin, dopamine) or a growth factor (brain-derived neurotrophic factor) that is involved in neural activity of some form.

Neuron

A neuron is a very specialized, impulse-conducting nerve cell. Although it is similar to

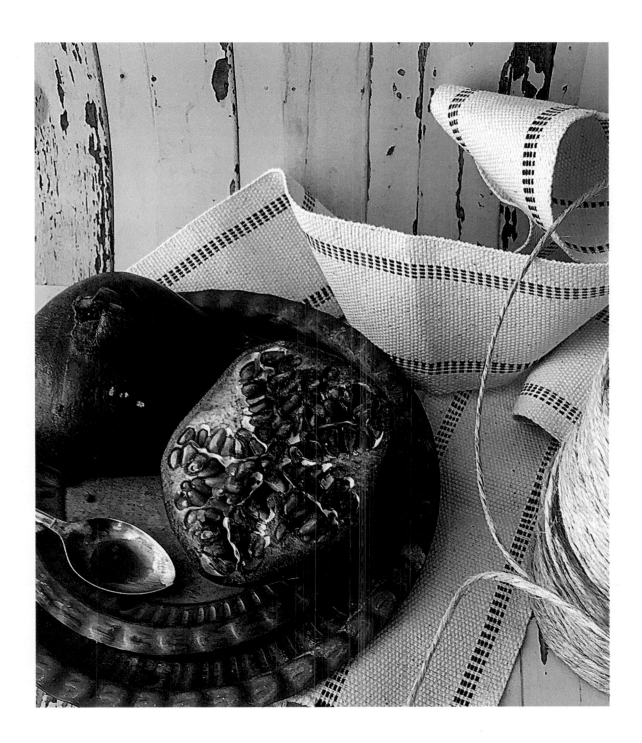

other cells in the body, it has a specialized way of transmitting information through the brain using electrochemical impulses. Neurons also contain specialized structures called axons and dendrites, which allow them to transmit and receive information very effectively.

Neuroplasticity

The ability of the brain to change and adapt is called neuroplasticity. The physical structure of the brain changes, much like soft plastic changes shape when it is exposed to external pressure. A young brain naturally has more 'plasticity' as it is developing and gaining skills, but all brains regardless of age can change and adapt as experience and learning imprints itself onto brain cells.

Neurotoxin

Any chemical that is harmful to neurons is called a neurotoxin. Neurotoxins can be found in many forms, such as in a gas, food additives or heavy metals. Even water can contain neurotoxins, such as chlorine and aluminium.

Neurotransmission

When a nerve impulse moves down an axon into a synapse, it is transmitting information via neurotransmitters. This process is called neurotransmission.

Neurotrophins

The family of proteins that promote the development, maintenance, survival and function of neurons. Brain-derived neurotrophic factor (BDNF) is a neurotrophin.

Noradrenaline

Noradrenaline, also known as norepinephrine, is a hormone released in the adrenal glands. It functions as a neurotransmitter and is also used in drug form to raise blood pressure. It is involved in focus and concentration.

Omega-3 fatty acids

These oils are called omega-3 fatty acids because they have a double bond at the third carbon atom along from the omega end of the fatty acid molecule.

Omega-6 fatty acids

These oils are called omega-6 fatty acids because they have a double bond at the sixth carbon atom along from the omega end of the fatty acid molecule.

Persistent organic pollutant (POP)

POPs are chemicals that are hazardous to our health and the environment. They are resistant to natural biodegradation or breakdown and tend to remain in our environment for a very long time. Many of them were created during the huge industrial boom after World War II. They can accumulate in the body, due to eating animals and products that contain them. They are fat-soluble so are incorporated into our fatty cell membranes and fat cells, hampering optimal cellular activity. The endocrine and reproductive system as well as the central nervous system are particularly susceptible to their toxic effects.

Phenylethylamine (PEA)

Phenylethylamine is an amine and neurotransmitter that resembles amphetamine in structure. PEA is found in high levels in chocolate, as well as in many cheeses and red wine.

Phospholipids (PLs)

A phospholipid is a fat molecule that has a glycerol backbone and is attached to a phosphorus atom with two fatty acids. They are the second major class of lipids found in the body and are found in all cell membranes.

Phytonutrients

These are natural chemicals found in plants thought to be beneficial to human health. Fruits, vegetables, legumes, grains, nuts and seeds, as well as herbs, teas and spices are known to contain phytonutrients.

Pituitary gland

The pituitary gland is the master endocrine gland in the brain. It secretes adrenocorticotropic hormone (ACTH), reproductive hormones, growth hormone, as well as other hormones that regulate various activities. The secretion of all these hormones is regulated by the hypothalamus, which stores them for future release.

Polyunsaturated fatty acids (PUFAs)

A polyunsaturated fatty acid is a fat molecule that has more than one double bond. EFAs are all polyunsaturated fats. They have between 18 and 22 carbon atoms. All PUFAs are also EFAs.

Prebiotics

Prebiotics are specific, non-digestible or partially digestible carbohydrates that feed probiotics. By promoting the growth of the helpful bacteria in our digestive system, they help to keep our digestive system working efficiently. They can be found in supplement form.

Probiotics

Probiotics are good bacteria, which ensure optimal absorption and digestion of nutrients in our digestive tract, as well as elimination of waste from our digestive system. When introduced into our body via oral supplementation, they can either replace or add to the beneficial bacteria already present in our digestive tract.

Progesterone

Progesterone is one of a group of hormones that maintain the natural course of pregnancy and the menstrual cycle of childbearing women. It is also used as a method of contraception and to regulate hormones when perimenopause or menopause causes hormone imbalance. Environmental oestrogens from meat, milk, plastics and pesticides dilute natural progesterone.

feed
your
brain

Prostaglandins

Prostaglandins (PGs) are hormone-like compounds that are produced from essential fatty acids (EFAs) within cell membranes. They are a subfamily of the eicosanoids. They are very potent but have a short life, which is why EFAs have to be replenished regularly. They have important functions in the human body and are found in most organs and tissues.

Rapid eye movement (REM) sleep

REM sleep is a specific type of sleep that occurs at regular intervals during the night. Your eyes move rapidly underneath your eyelids, hence the name, and your brain is producing images that you will recall as dreams. Your pulse and breathing rate goes up, as does your physical movement although muscles are paralyzed to a degree to protect you from acting on your dreams and thereby hurting yourself.

Ribonucleic acid (RNA)

RNA is a compound present in the nucleus of all living cells. It is a messenger, carrying information from DNA, which controls the synthesis of proteins.

S-adenosylmethionine (SAMe)

SAMe is a naturally occurring chemical in the body involved in the synthesis of amino acids. It can also be produced commercially. The body uses SAMe to make specific compounds that are used to manage pain and mood among other things.

Salicylates

Salicylates occur naturally in many plants, acting as a natural pesticide against disease and insects. They are produced commercially, with aspirin being the best known. Some people are sensitive to them and react with headaches, behaviour challenges, anxiety, depression and sleep disturbances.

Saturated fatty acids (SFAs)

A saturated fatty acid (SFA) is a fat molecule that has no double bonds. It can have between two and 24 carbon atoms in its molecular chain. They are literally 'saturated' with hydrogen atoms, so there can be no double carbon-to-carbon bonds in these molecules. Saturated fatty acids can be either short-, medium- or long-chain.

Serine

Serine is an amino acid found in most proteins. It forms part of the compound called phosphotidylserine, which is an important phospholipid, involved in membrane structure and myelin, which is the insulation that surrounds axons.

Synapse

The connections between neurons are known as synapses. Messages are sent between neurons from the synaptic 'cleft' or membrane, using compounds called neurotransmitters.

Tartrazine

Tartrazine is a chemical synthesized from coal

tar. It may have salicylate properties, leading to hay fever symptoms as well as some skin conditions. It also causes zinc loss via the kidneys, and has been linked to hyperactivity in children.

Taurine

Taurine is an amino acid made from cysteine and methionine. It plays an important role in the metabolism of fats (fatty acids).

Testosterone

Testosterone is the primary male hormone regulating the growth, development and maintenance of sexual organs and function. As testosterone levels fall with age, supplementing with it can counter some age-related hormonal changes.

Trans fatty acids (TFAs)

A TFA molecule is a damaged fat molecule. A TFA is formed either through a process called hydrogenation or through heating a fat/oil. The fat molecule moves around a double carbon bond and the hydrogen atom jumps across the double bond to the other side. This jump across the carbon bond can occur at more than one double carbon bond, leading to more damaged fat molecules. The body and brain do not recognize these damaged fats and they interfere with optimal cellular function.

Triglycerides

Triglycerides are the most abundant type of fat in the body and are made up of various combinations of different types of fatty acids. They have a glycerol backbone, to which three (tri) fatty acids are attached. The type of fatty acid (ie. saturated, monounsaturated, polyunsaturated or a combination), will determine whether they lead to health or disease.

Tyramine

Tyramine is an amino acid that occurs naturally in the body and is found in certain foods. It helps to regulate blood pressure. If taking a monoamine oxidase inhibitor (MAOI) you will need to avoid consuming foods that contain tyramine.

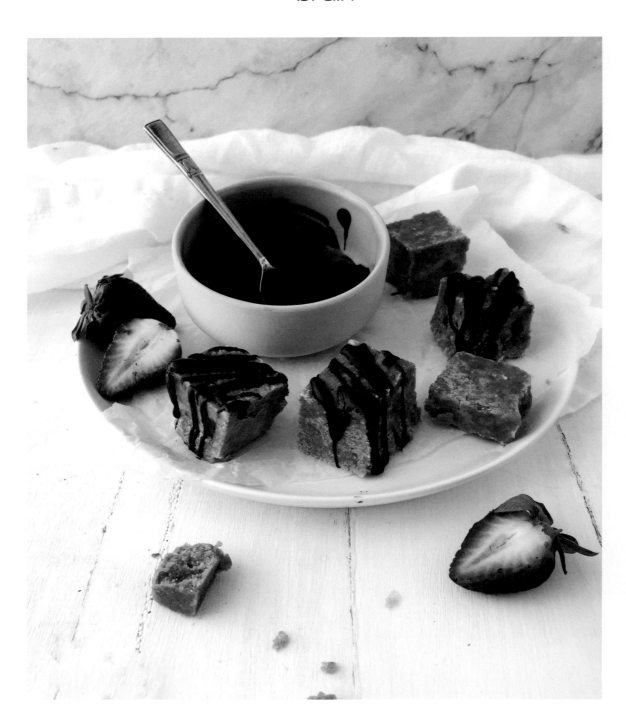

Resources

Exercise

www.mayoclinic.org/healthy-living/fitness/in-depth/fitness/art-20047624

www.oxygenmag.com/article/27-ways-to-stay-motivated-6526

Far infrared saunas

www.greatsaunas.com/info/40-facts-for-far-infrared-saunas.cfm

'Smart' computer games

www.lumosity.com

www.brainhq.com

Volunteering

www.do-it.org/news/welcome (UK)

www.createthegood.org/about (USA)

www.govolunteer.com.au (Australia)

Sleep challenges

www.sleepfoundation.org (USA)

www.sleepcouncil.org.uk/2012/03/sleep-well-feel-well (UK)

www.sleephealthfoundation.org.au (Australia)

Stress

www.slowmagazine.com.au (Australia)

HeartMath is a unique way to reduce stress levels using technology and science to align the heart, mind and emotions: www.heartmath.com

Manage stress using Neurofeedback: www.isnr.org

Practitioners

American Academy of Environmental Medicine to find a qualified practitioner in your area: www.aaemonline.org

The Australasian College of Nutritional and Environmental Medicine – find a practitioner in your area: www.acnem.org

The Brain BioCentre (United Kingdom): www.foodforthebrain.org/brain-bio-centre.aspx

Micronutrient assessments including MTHFR testing
SpectraCell Laboratories offer comprehensive nutritional testing programmes (USA):
www.spectracell.com/patients/products
www.greatplainslaboratory.com/home/eng/food_allergy_igg.asp

Certified organic skin, body and hair care products
www.miessence.com
www.muktiorganics.com
www.acureorganics.com
www.thedivinecompany.com
www.intelligentnutrients.com
www.natulique.com

Supplements
Essential fatty acids, digestive enzymes and probiotics (America and Canada):
www.florahealth.com/home_ca.cfm
Essential fatty acids (Australia): www.ntphealthproducts.com/index.html
Essential fatty acids (United Kingdom): www.udoschoice.co.uk/products
www.metagenics.com.au (Australia)
www.metagenics.com (United States)
www.metagenics.eu (Europe)
www.lef.org
www.mediherb.com
www.coconutmagic.com

Reasons to buy organic
www.organicconsumers.org/old_articles/organlink.php
www.prevention.com/food/healthy-eating-tips/top-reasons-choose-organic-foods
www.organic.org/articles/showarticle/article-206
www.austorganic.com

Resources

Sustainable seafood

Australia's sustainable seafood guide: www.sustainableseafood.org.au

Guides to sustainable fish around the world: www.slowfood.com/slowfish/pagine/eng/pagina.lasso?-id_pg=94

Green choices for home building, maintenance and cleaning

www.epa.gov/greenhomes/protectingyourhealth.htm (USA)

www.yourhome.gov.au/appendices/healthy-home (Australia)

www.earthfirst.net.au (Australia)

www.aecb.net (United Kingdom)

Food dyes, additives and behavioural challenges

Center for Science in the Public Interest (www.cspinet.org) features articles about food dyes and behavioural challenges (USA)

www.additivealert.com.au (Australia)

www.food.gov.uk/safereating/chemsafe/additivesbranch/enumberlist (United Kingdom)

www.foodstandards.gov.au (Australia)

www.fedupwithfoodadditives.info (Australia)

www.chemicalmaze.com

Mercury filling removal

www.iaomt.org/safe-removal-amalgam-fillings/

Further information

www.ion.ac.uk

www.udoerasmus.com

www.sciencebasedmedicine.org/igg-food-intolerance-tests-what-does-the-science-say

www.fluoridealert.org/issues/water/

www.johnleemd.com/

lpi.oregonstate.edu/

www2.epa.gov/international-cooperation/persistent-organic-pollutants-global-issue-global-response#pops

www.sustainweb.org

www.ancient-minerals.com

International Olive Council: www.internationaloliveoil.org

North American Olive Oil Association (NAAOA): www.naooa.org

SeaWeb: www.seaweb.org/resources/briefings/atsalmon.php

Acknowledgements

This book only exists because of the wonderful men and women who have dedicated their lives to discovering more about our fantastic brain and what it needs to function optimally. I have had the wonderful privilege of reading the journal articles and books that many of these well-respected researchers have written. I have met some of them in person too, and because we live in a virtual world, I have met even more online! It has also been an unexpected surprise to find that many of them have gone the extra mile for me by suggesting other journal articles and books to delve into. Although this isn't an exhaustive list by far, my sincere thanks go to the following people:

Dr Abraham Hoffer, a visionary who laid the foundation for tackling mental health challenges with nutrients. Although Dr Hoffer has now passed away, his research and the people he inspired have been immensely valuable to me.

Dr Udo Erasmus, a pioneer in the use of fats and oils for optimal health, who is always willing to answer my questions.

Professor Michael Crawford, the Director of the Institute of Brain Chemistry and Human Nutrition at London Metropolitan University and a consultant for the World Health Organization, who has been involved in brain research for over five decades, and who has been extremely helpful in providing research papers as well as his time to discuss the enormous mental health challenges that we are facing as a species.

Professor Stephen Schoenthaler from California State University who pioneered nutrition and behaviour research in juvenile detention centres decades ago and who has been intimately involved in investigating the impact of poor food choices and behaviour. He has been helpful in explaining how the research into nutrition and the brain has advanced over the decades.

Professor Richard Wurtman from MIT, who has been actively involved in research into preventing cognitive decline and who has been extremely helpful to me, providing his research papers and insightful thoughts about nutrition and the brain, especially the ageing brain.

Dr Bruce Ames, a pioneer in mitochondria research.

Dr Vernon Barnes, who researches how meditation heals the brain.

David Ogilvie, who has studied the changes in soil nutrient levels over the past few decades.

Dr Dharma Singh Khalsa, a pioneer in nutrition and healing the brain.

Dr Daniel Amen, a pioneer in using brain imaging to understand mental health challenges.

Dr David Perlmutter, a pioneer in nutrition and the ageing brain.

Acknowledgements

Professor Felice Jacka at Deakin University, who has been investigating nutrition and children's mental health for a number of years and who is particularly interested in the connection between depression and dietary choices.

Professor David Benton, who has researched the effects of specific nutrients on mood for many decades.

Dr Walter Willett, the head of the Department of Nutrition at Harvard School of Public Health, who has been researching nutrient intake and health for over five decades.

A very big thank you to the team at Exisle! Although writing a book is a fabulous experience, it's also quite lonely and you've made it much less so with your great ideas, support, patience and hand-holding!

A special thank you to Kathy Archer who has a busy practice and life, but still took the time to read my manuscript and comment on its content and usefulness!

A special thank you to Maryanne Haarvoor, who helped me to start the gluten-free baking journey, and whose creativity sparked the origin of many a healthy family meal.

And thank you to Vanessa Russell from Raspberry Creative for the mouthwatering photographs and to Luke McManus for the gorgeous graphics.

And finally, my family, who have been tolerant of the not-so-tasty experiments that have come out of my kitchen! A special thank you to my husband, who has supported me on this adventure of discovery and encouraged me to share its findings with others!

A very special thank you to my mother who taught me about the importance of healthy food long before it was fashionable; who made sprouts long before they were fashionable, or easy to make; and who has believed in my message and encouraged me at every turn!

References

Introduction

Sabia S. et al. Health behaviors from early to late midlife as predictors of cognitive function: The Whitehall II study. *Am J Epidemiol*. 2009 Aug 15;170(4):428–37.

Akbaraly T et al. Does overall diet in midlife predict future aging phenotypes? A cohort study. *Am J Med*. 2013 May;126(5):411–419.

Loef M and Walach H. The combined effects of healthy lifestyle behaviors on all cause mortality: a systematic review and meta-analysis. *Prev Med*. 2012 Sep;55(3):163–70.

www.psychology.org.au/inpsych/2012/august/crowe/ (accessed 10 December 2014).

www.blackdoginstitute.org.au/docs/Factsandfig uresaboutmentalhealthand-mooddisorders.pdf (accessed 2 December 2014).

www.healthdata.org/research-article/global-burden-disease-attributable-mental-and-substance-use-disorders-findings (accessed 5 September 2015).

www.madinamerica.com/2013/07/why-the-dramat-ic-rise-of-mental-illness-diseasing-normal-behav-iors-drug-adverse-effects-and-a-peculiar-rebellion/ (accessed 7 September 2015).

www.calmclinic.com/anxiety/anxiety-disorder-sta-tistics (accessed 8 December 2014).

www.nimh.nih.gov/health/statistics/index.shtml (accessed 28 November 2014).

http://uk.reuters.com/article/2013/07/24/us-brain-costs-idUKBRE96N1I120130724 (accessed 16 September 2015).

www.mentalhealth.org.uk/content/assets/PDF/campaigns/MHF-Business-case-for-MH-research-Nov2010.pdf (accessed 10 November 2014).

Chapter 1: Sweat, Sleep, Sex and Stress — What they mean to your brain

Cohen, GD. *The Mature Mind: the positive power of the aging brain*. Basic Books, Cambridge, MA, 2006.

Small, G. *The Memory Prescription: Dr Gary Small's 14-Day Plan to Keep Your Brain and Body Young*. Hyperion Books, New York, 2004.

Buzan, T. *Age-proof Your Brain: sharpen your memory in 7 days*. Thorsons, London, 2009.

Brain rules – *12 principles for surviving and thriving at work, home, and school*. Medina J. Pear Press Pub. Seattle. 2008.

Wilson RS, Krueger KR, Arnold SE, Schneider JA, Kelly JF, Barnes LL, Tang Y, Bennett DA. Loneliness and risk of Alzheimer disease. *Arch Gen Psychiatry*. 2007 Feb;64(2):234–40.

Wilson RS et al. Negative social interactions and risk of mild cognitive impairment in old age. *Neuropsychology*. 2015 Jul;29(4):561–70.

Stephan Y et al. Association of personality with physical, social, and mental activities across the lifespan: findings from US and French samples. *Br J Psychol*. 2014 Nov;105(4):564–80.

Schwartz ET and Holtorf K. Hormones in wellness and disease prevention: common practices, current state of the evidence, and questions for the future. *Prim Care*. 2008 Dec;35(4):669–705.

Holtorf K. The bioidentical hormone debate: are bioidentical hormones (estradiol, estriol, and progesterone) safer or more efficacious than commonly used synthetic versions in hormone replacement therapy? Postgrad Med. 2009 Jan;121(1):73–85.

Sweat/exercise

Doidge N. *The Brain That Changes Itself*, Scribe Publications, Carlton North, 2007.

Cotman CW et al. Exercise enhances and protects brain function. *Exerc Sport Sci Rev*. 2002 Apr;30(2):75–9.

Berchtold NC et al. Exercise and time-dependant

benefits to learning and memory. *Neuroscience.* 2010 May 19;167(3):588–97.

Geda YE et al. Physical exercise, aging, and mild cognitive impairment: a population-based study. *Arch Neurol.* 2010 Jan;67(1):80–6.

Horstman J. *The Scientific American Brave New Brain.* Jossey-Bass, San Francisco, 2010.

Emoto K. Dendrite remodeling in development and disease. *Dev Growth Differ.* 2011 Apr;53(3):277–86.

Cotman CW et al. Exercise: a behavioural intervention to enhance brain health and plasticity. *Trends Neurosci.* 2002 Jun;25(6):295–301.

Kramer AF et al. Capitalizing on cortical plasticity: influence of physical activity on cognition and brain function. *Trends Cogn Sci.* 2007 Aug;11(8):342–8.

Bjørnebekk A et al. The antidepressant effect of running is associated with increased hippocampal cell proliferation. *Int J Neuropsychopharmacol.* 2005 Sep;8(3):357–68.

Hillman CH, et al. Be smart, exercise your heart: exercise effects on brain and cognition. *Nat Rev Neurosci.* 2008 Jan;9(1):58–65.

Ratey JJ and Hagerman E. *Spark: the revolutionary new science of exercise and the brain.* Little Brown and Company, New York. 2008.

Pinilla FG. The impact of diet and exercise on brain plasticity and disease. *Nutr Health.* 2006;18(3):277–84.

Dietrich MO et al. Exercise induced synaptogenesis in the hippocampus is dependent on UCP2-regulated mitochondrial adaptation. *J Neurosci.* 2008 Oct 15;28(42):10766–71.

Yamada K et al. Role for brain-derived neurotrophic factor in learning and memory. *Life Sci.* 2002 Jan 4;70(7):735–44.

Balaratnasingam S et al. Brain Derived Neurotrophic Factor: a novel neurotrophin involved in psychiatric and neurological disorders. *Pharmacol Ther.* 2012 Apr;134(1):116–24.

Victoroff J. Heal the heart, the mind will follow.

Harvard Heart Letter 2005 Jul;15(11):1–2.

Victoroff J. *Saving Your Brain: the revolutionary plan to boost brain power, improve memory, and protect yourself against aging and Alzheimer's.* Bantam Books, Milsons Point, 2002.

Van Praag H. Exercise and the brain: something to chew on. *Trends Neurosci.* 2009 May;32(5):283–90.

Deslandes A. The biological clock keeps ticking, but exercise may turn it back. *Arq neuropsiquiatr.* 2013 Feb;71(2) 113–8.

Lozada M et al. Beneficial effects of human altruism. *J Theor Biol.* 2011 Nov 21;289:12–6.

Mahncke HW et al. Brain plasticity and functional losses in the aged: scientific bases for a novel intervention. *Prog Brain Res.* 2006;157:81–109.

Sleep

Czeisler CA et al. Sleep and circadian rhythms in humans. *Cold Spring Harb Symp Quant Biol.* 2007;72:579–97.

Wright KP Jr et al. Sleep and wakefulness out of phase with internal biological time impairs learning in humans. *J Cogn Neurosci.* 2006 Apr;18(4):508–21.

Malik SW et al. Sleep deprivation. *Prim Care.* 2005 Jun;32(2):475–90.

Havekes R et al. The impact of sleep deprivation on neuronal and glial signalling pathways important for memory and synaptic plasticity. *Cell Signal.* 2012 Jun;24(6):1251–60.

Talamini LM et al. Sleep directly following learning benefits consolidation of spatial associative memory. *Learn Mem.* 2008 Apr 3;15(4):233–7.

Van Dongen HP et al. The cumulative cost of additional wakefulness: dose-response effects on neurobehavioral functions and sleep physiology from chronic sleep restriction and total sleep deprivation. *Sleep.* 2003 Mar 15;26(2):117–26.

Perlmutter D and Colman C. *The Better Brain Book: the best tools for improving memory and sharpness and preventing aging of the brain.* Berkeley

Publishing Group, New York. 2004.

Oztürk L et al. Effects of 48 hours sleep deprivation on human immune profile. *Sleep Res Online*. 1999;2(4):107–11.

Jakobson Ramin C. *Carved in Sand: when attention fails and memory fades in midlife*. Harper Luxe, New York. 2007.

Sapolsky RM. *Why Zebras Don't Get Ulcers: the acclaimed guide to stress, stress-related diseases and coping*, 3rd edition. Henry Holt and Company, LLC New York, 2004.

Stickgold R et al. Sleep-dependant memory consolidation and reconsolidation. *Sleep Med*. 2007 Jun;8(4):331–43.

Walker MP et al. Sleep, memory, and plasticity. *Annu Rev Psychol*. 2006;57:139–66.

Ellenbogen JM et al. Interfering with theories of sleep and memory: sleep, declarative memory, and associative interference. *Curr Biol*. 2006 Jul 11;16(13):1290–4.

Vertes RP. Memory consolidation in sleep: dream or reality. *Neuron*. 2004 Sep 30;44(1):135–48.

Stevenson R. 1892. A Chapter on Dreams. *Selected Essays of Robert Louis Stevenson*.

http://etc.usf.edu/lit2go/110/selected-essays-of-robert-louis-stevenson/5111/a-chapter-on-dreams/ (accessed 3 November 2014).

Barry Miles. *Paul McCartney: many years from now*. Henry Holt, New York, 1997.

Roberts RM. *Serendipity: accidental discoveries in science*. Wiley, New York, 1989.

A'Lelia Bundles. *On Her Own Ground: The life and times of Madam CJ Walker*, Scribner, New York, 2001.

Kaempffert W (ed.). *A Popular History of American Invention, Vol. II*. Scribner's Sons, New York, 1924.

Jack Nicklaus as told to a *San Francisco Chronicle* reporter, 27 June 1964.

Singh Khalsa D and Stauth C. *The Mind Miracle*.

Arrow Books, London, 1998.

Gottlieb DJ et al. Association of usual sleep duration with hypertension: the Sleep Heart Health Study. *Sleep*. 2006 Aug 1;29(8):1009–14.

Chaput JP et al. The association between sleep duration and weight gain in adults: a 6-year prospective study from the Quebec Family Study. *Sleep*. 2008 Apr 1;31(4):517–23.

Adámkova V et al. Association between duration of the sleep and body weight. *Physiol Res*. 2009 58:Suppl 1:S27–S31.

Trenell MI et al. Sleep and metabolic control: waking to a problem? *Clin Exp Pharmcol Physiol*. 2007 Jan–Feb;34(1–2):1–9.

Meerlo P et al. New neurons in the adult brain: the role of sleep and consequence of sleep loss. *Sleep Med Rev*. 2009 Jun;13(3):187–94.

Xie L et al. Sleep drives metabolite clearance from the adult brain. *Science*. 2013 Oct 18;342(6156):373–7.

Sex

Michaud E with Bain J. Sleep to be sexy, smart and slim. *Readers Digest*, 2008.

Komisaruk BR et al. Functional MRI of the brain during orgasm in women. *Annu Rev Sex Res*. 2005;16:62–86.

Grewen KM et al. Warm partner contact is related to lower cardiovascular reactivity. *Behav Med*. 2003 Fall;29(3):123–30.

Lindau ST et al. A study of sexuality and health among older adults in the United States. *N Engl J Med*. 2007 Aug 23;357(8):762–74.

Brody S. Blood pressure reactivity to stress is better for people who recently had penile-vaginal intercourse than for people who had other or no sexual activity. *Biol Psychol*. 2006 Feb;71(2):214–22.

Glenville M. *The New Natural Alternatives to HRT*. Kyle Cathie Limited, London, 2007.

References

Schumaker SA et al. Estrogen plus progestin and the incidence of dementia and mild cognitive impairment in postmenopausal women: the Women's Health Initiative Memory Study: a randomised controlled trial. *JAMA*, 2003 May 28;289(20):2651–62.

Somers S. *Ageless: the naked truth about bioidentical hormones*. Crown Publishing Group, New York, 2006.

Weber M et al. Memory complaints and memory performance in the menopausal transition. *Menopause*. 2009 Jul–Aug;16(4):694–700.

Stress

Talbott S. *The Cortisol Connection: why stress makes you fat and ruins your health and what you can do about it*. Hunter House Publishers, California, 2002.

Smith MA. Hippocampal vulnerability to stress and aging: possible role of neurotrophic factors. *Behav Brain Res*. 1996 Jun;78(1):25–36.

Virtanen M et al. Long working hours and cognitive function: the Whitehall II study. *Am J Epidemiol*. 2009 Mar 1;169(5):596–605.

Dusek JA et al. Mind-body medicine: a model of the comparative impact of the acute stress and relaxation responses. *Minn Med* 2009 May;92(5):47–50.

Chatta R et al. Effect of yoga on cognitive functions in climacteric syndrome: a randomised control study. *BJOG*. 2008 Jul;115(8):991–1000.

Epel E, et al. Can meditation slow rate of cellular aging? Cognitive stress, mindfulness, and telomeres. *Ann N Y Acad Sci*. 2009 Aug;1172:34–53.

Braverman, ER. *The Healing Nutrients Within*. Basic Health Publications, California, 2003.

Cabot S. *Magnesium: the miracle mineral*. WHAS, Australia, 2007.

Perlmutter, D and Colman C. *The Better Brain Book: the best tools for improving memory and sharpness and preventing aging of the brain*. Penguin, New York, 2004.

Ohayon MM et al. Place of chronic insomnia in the course of depressive and anxiety disorders. *J Psychiatr Res*. 2003 Jan–Feb;37(1):9–15.

Logan, AC. *The Brain Diet*. Cumberland House Publishing, Tennessee, 2007.

Epel E et al. Stress may add bite to appetite in women: a laboratory study of stress-induced cortisol and eating behaviour. *Psychoneuroendocrinology*. 2001 Jan;26(1):37–49.

Corsica JA et al. Carbohydrate craving: a double-blind, placebo-controlled test of the self-medication hypothesis. *Eat Behav*. 2008 Dec;9(4):447–54.

Chiesa A. Zen meditation: an integration of current evidence. *J Altern Complement Med*. 2009 May;15(5):585–92.

Vestergaard-Poulsen P et al. Long-term meditation is associated with increased gray matter density in the brain stem. *Neuroreport*. 2009 Jan 28;20(2):170–4.

Chapter 2: What food intolerances do to your brain

Logan AC. *The Brain Diet*. Cumberland House Publishing, Tennessee, 2007.

Perlmutter D and Colman C. *The Better Brain Book: the best tools for improving memory and sharpness and preventing aging of the brain*. Berkeley Publishing Group, New York. 2004.

Gupta R et al. Burden of allergic disease in the UK: secondary analyses of national databases. *Clin Exp Allergy*. 2004 Apr;34(4):5206.

Barnard N. *Breaking the Food Addiction: the hidden reasons behind food cravings and 7 steps to end them naturally*. St Martins Press, New York, 2003.

Holford P and Braley J *Hidden Food allergies: is what you eat making you ill?* Piatkus London, 2005.

Breakey J. *Are You Food Sensitive?* CE Breakey Medical Pty Ltd, 1998.

Buist R. *Food Chemical Sensitivity*. Harper and Row, London, 1986.

Rippere V. Some varieties of food intolerance in psychiatric patients: an overview. *Nutr Health.* 1984;3(3):125–36.

Hall K. Allergy of the nervous system: a review. *Ann Allergy.* 1976 Jan;36(1):49–64.

Haynes, AJ. Chapter 10: The effect of food intolerance and allergy on mood and behaviour in *Nutrition and Mental Health: a handbook* by Watts, M (ed). Pavilion, Brighton, 2009.

Addolorato G et al. Anxiety and depression: a common feature of health care seeking patients with bowel syndrome and food allergy. *Hepatogastroenterology.* 1998 Sep–Oct;45(23):1559–64.

Marshall PS. Allergy and depression: a neurochemical threshold model of the relation between the illnesses. *Psychol Bull.* 1993 Jan;113(1):23–43.

Karakula-Juchnowicz H et al. The role of IgG hypersensitivity in the pathogenesis and therapy of depressive disorders. *Nutr Neurosci.* 2014 Sep 30 [Epub ahead of print].

Pfeiffer CC. *Nutrition and Mental Illness.* Healing Arts Press, Rochester, 1987.

Geary A. *Food and Mood Handbook: find relief at last from depression, anxiety, PMS, cravings and mood swings.* Thorsons, London, 2001.

Campbell-McBride N. Chapter 7: Gut and psychology syndrome (GAP syndrome or GAPS™) in *Nutrition and Mental Health: a handbook* by Watts, M (ed). Pavilion, Brighton, 2009.

Spangler R et al. Opiate-like effects of sugar on gene expression in reward areas of the brain. *Brain Res Mol Brain Res.* 2004 May 19;124(2):134–42.

Hazum E et al. Morphine in cow and human milk: could dietary morphine constitute a ligand for specific morphine (mu) receptors? *Science.* 1981 Aug 28;213(4511):1010–2.

Meisel H. Biochemical properties of peptides encrypted in bovine milk proteins. *Curr Med Chem.* 2005;12(16):1905–19.

Braly J and Hoggan R. *Dangerous Grains.* Avery Books, New York, 2002.

Korn D. *Wheat-free, Worry-free: the art of happy, healthy, gluten-free living.* Hay House, California, 2002.

Ford R. *Full of It! The shocking truth about gluten: The brain-grain connection.* RRS Global Pub, New Zealand, 2006.

Hadjivassiliou M et al. Headache and CNS white matter abnormalities associated with gluten sensitivity. *Neurology.* 2001 Feb 13;56(3):385–8.

Perlmutter D. *Grain Brain.* Little Brown and Company, New York, 2013.

Lurie Y et al. Celiac disease diagnosed in the elderly. *J Clin Gastroenterol.* 2008 Jan;429(1):59–61.

Perlmutter D and Loberg K. *Brain Maker: the power of gut microbes to heal and protect your brain — for life.* Hodder & Stoughton Ltd, London, 2015.

Bested AC et al. Intestinal microbiota, probiotics and mental health: from Metchnikoff to modern advances: Part I — autointoxication revisited. *Gut Pathogens.* 2013 Mar 18;5(1):5.

Bested AC et al. Intestinal microbiota, probiotics and mental health: from Metchnikoff to modern advances: Part II — contemporary contextual research. *Gut Pathogens.* 2013 Mar 14;5(1):3.

Bested AC et al. Intestinal microbiota, probiotics and mental health: from Metchnikoff to modern advances: Part III — convergence toward clinical trials. *Gut Pathogens.* 2013 Mar 16;5(1):4.

Dinan TG et al. Regulation of the stress response by the gut microbiota: Implications for psychoneuroendocrinology. *Psychoneuroendocrinology.* 2012 Sept;37(9):1369–78.

Dinan TG et al. Probiotics in the treatment of depression: science or science fiction? *Aust NZ J Psychiatry.* 2011 Dec;45(12):1023–5.

Foster JA et al. Gut–brain axis: how the microbiome influences anxiety and depression. *Trends in Neurosciences,* 2013 May;36(5):305–12.

Schmidt K et al. Prebiotic intake reduces the waking

cortisol response and alters emotional bias in healthy volunteers. *Psychopharmacology* (Berl). 2014 Dec 3 [Epub ahead of print].

Fond G et al. The 'psychomicrobiotic': targeting microbiota in major psychiatric disorders: a systematic review. *Pathol Biol* (Paris). 2014 Nov 2 [Epub ahead of print].

Bray GA. Afferent signals regulating food intake. *Proc Nutr Soc*. 2000 Aug;59(3):373–84.

Jacobsen MB et al. Relation between food provocation and systemic immune activation in patients with food intolerance. *Lancet*. 2000 Jul 29;356(9227)400–1.

Mullin GE et al. Testing for food reactions: the good, the bad, and the ugly. *Nutr Clin Pract*. 2010 Apr;25(2):192–8.

Chapter 3: Why food additives are bad for your brain

Haas EM and Levin B. *Staying Healthy with Nutrition: the complete guide to diet and nutritional medicine*. Celestial Arts, Berkeley, 2006.

Lonky S and Deitsch RJ. *Invisible Killers: the truth about environmental genocide*. IK Enterprises, USA, 2007.

Schlosser E. *Fast Food Nation: what the all-American meal is doing to the world*. Penguin Books, London, 2002.

Contreras F. *Health in the 21st Century: will doctors survive?* Interpacific Press, California, 1997.

Baillie-Hamilton, P. *Stop the 21st Century Killing You*. Vermilion Books, London, 2005.

Steinman D. *Diet for a poisoned planet: how to choose safe foods for you and your family*. Ballantine Books, New York, 1990.

Robbins, J. *Diet for a New America: how your food choices affect your health, happiness and the future of life on earth* 2nd edn. HJ Kramer Inc, California, 1998.

Skurray G. *Decoding Food Additives: a comprehensive guide to food additive codes*. Hachette Australia, Sydney, 2005.

Tong M et al. Nitrosamine exposure causes insulin resistance diseases: relevance to Type 2 Diabetes Mellitus, Non-Alcoholic Steatohepatitis, and Alzheimer's disease. *J Alzheimers Dis*. 2009;17(4):327–44.

Dietrich M et al. A review: dietary and endogenously formed N-nitroso compounds and risk of childhood brain tumors. *Cancer Causes Control*. 2005 Aug;16(6):619–35.

Eady J. *Additive Alert: your guide to safer shopping*. Additive Alert Pty Ltd, Mullaloo, WA, 2004.

Blaylock RL. *Excitotoxins: the taste that kills*. Health Press, Sante Fe, 1997.

Statham B. *The Chemical Maze Shopping Companion: your guide to food additives and cosmetic ingredients* 3rd edn. Possibility.com, Neerim South, Australia, 2006.

Bellisle F et al. Intense sweeteners, energy intake and the control of body weight. *Eur J Clin Nutr*. 2007 Jun;61(6):691–700.

Tsakiris S et al. The effect of aspartame metabolites on human erythrocyte membrane acetylcholinesterase activity. *Pharmacol Res*. 2006 Jan;53(1):1–5.

Lau K et al. Synergistic interactions between commonly used food additives in a developmental neurotoxicity test. *Toxicol Sci*. 2006 March; 90(1):178–87.

Haveland-Smith RB et al. Screening of food dyes for genotoxic activity. *Food Cosmet Toxicol*. 1980 Jun;18(3):215–21.

Kobylewski S et al. Toxicology of food dyes. *Int J Occup Environ Health*. 2012 Jul–Sep;18(3):220–46.

Stejskal, V. Chapter 4: The effect of mercury on the body and brain in *Nutrition and Mental Health: a handbook*. Watts, M (ed). Pavilion, Brighton, 2009.

Ritter L et al. Persistent organic pollutants: an assessment report on: DDT, aldrin, dieldrin, endrin, chlordane, heptachlor, hexachlorobenzene, mirex, toxaphene, polychlorinated biphenyls, dioxins and furans. Prepared for The International

Programme on Chemical Safety (IPCS) within the framework of the Inter-Organization Programme for the Sound Management of Chemicals (IOMC). Canadian Network of Toxicology Centers, Guelph, Ontario, 1995. www.who.int/ipcs/assessment/en/pcs_95_39_2004_05_13.pdf

Holtcamp W. Obesogens: an environmental link to obesity. *Environ Health Perspect*. 2012 Feb;120(2):a62–8.

Grün F. Obesogens. *Curr Opin Endocrinol Diabetes Obes*. 2010 Oct;17(5):453–9.

Soto AM et al. Environmental causes of cancer: endocrine disruptors as carcinogens. *Nat Rev Endocrinol*. 2010 Jul;6(7):363–70.

Baillie-Hamilton PF. Chemical toxins: a hypothesis to explain the global obesity epidemic. *J Altern Complement Med*. 2002 Apr;8(2):185–92.

Smith R and Lourie B. *Slow Death By Rubber Duck: how the toxic chemistry of everyday life affects our health*. University of Queensland Press, Brisbane. 2009.

Grandjean P et al. Neurobehavioral effects of developmental toxicity. *Lancet Neurol*. 2014 Mar;13(3):330–8.

Chapter 4: The vitamins and minerals your brain needs

Winter A and Winter R. *Smart Food: diet and nutrition for maximum brain power*. ASJA Press, New York, 2007.

Davies S. 'The myth of the balanced diet.' Interview at Institute of Optimum Nutrition, UK, 1994.

https://fnic.nal.usda.gov/surveys-reports-and-research/food-and-nutrition-surveys/national-health-and-nutrition-examination (accessed 12 October 2015).

www.crnusa.org/benefits/files/02CRN-Benefits-Book-whoneeds.pdf (accessed 25 September 2015).

Moshfegh A, Goldman J and Cleveland L. *What We Eat In America, NHANES 2001–2002: usual nutrient intakes from food compared to dietary reference intakes*. US Department of Agriculture, Agriculture Research Service, 2005.

Murphy MM. Revising the daily values may affect food fortification and in turn nutrient intake adequacy. *J Nutr*. 2013 Dec;143(12):1999–2006.

Schauss AG. Suggested Optimum Nutrient Intake of Vitamins, Minerals, and Trace Elements in Pizzorno J and Murray MT (eds), *Textbook of Natural Medicine* 3rd edn. Vol 2:1275–1320. Churchill Livingstone/Elsevier, St Louis, 2006.

McGuire M and Beerman K. *Nutritional Sciences: from fundamentals to food*, 3rd edn. Wadsworth Cengage Learning, Belmont, California, 2011.

Holford P. *The New Optimum Nutrition Bible*. Crossing Press, London, 2005.

Bronstein AC et al. 2009 Annual Report of the American Association of Poison Control Center's National Poison Data System (NPDS): 27th Annual Report. *Clinical Toxicology*. 2010;48:979–1178. The full text article is available for free download at www.aapcc.org/annual-reports/

Neuhouser ML et al. Multivitamin use and risk of cancer and CVD in women's health initiative cohorts. *Arch Intern Med*. 2009;169(3):294–304.

Block G et al. Usage patterns, health and nutritional status of long-term multiple dietary supplement users: a cross-sectional study. *Nutr J*. 2007 Oct 24;6:30.

Xu Q et al. Multivitamin use and telomere length in women. *Am J Clin Nutr*. 2009 Jun;89(6):1857–63.

www.organic-center.org/reportfiles/Nutrient_Content_SSR_Executive_Summary_2008.pdf (accessed 12 September 2015).

Baillie-Hamilton P. *Stop the 21st Century Killing You*. Vermilion Books, London, 2005.

Victoroff J. *Saving Your Brain: the revolutionary plan to boost brain power, improve memory, and protect yourself against aging and Alzheimer's*. Bantam Books, Milsons Point, 2002.

Singh Khalsa D and Stauth C. *The Mind Miracle*.

References

Arrow Books, London, 1998.

Prasad C. *Nutritional Neuroscience: Nutrition, Brain and Behaviour* by Lieberman HR, Kanarek RB, Prasad C (eds). Taylor & Francis Group, Florida. 2005; chapters 13–18.

Solfrizzi V et al. The role of diet in cognitive decline. *Neural Transm.* 2003 Jan;110(1):96–110.

Polidori MC et al. High fruit and vegetable intake is positively correlated with antioxidant status and cognitive performance in healthy subjects. *J Alzheimers Dis.* 2009;17(4):921–7.

Vercambre MN et al. Long-term association of food and nutrient intakes with cognitive and functional decline: a 13-year follow-up study of elderly French women. *Br J Nutr.* 2009 Aug;102(3):419–27.

Oude Griep LM et al. Raw and processed fruit and vegetable consumption and 10-year stroke incidence in a population-based cohort study in the Netherlands. *Eur J Clin Nutr.* 2011 Jul;65(7):791–9.

Fehm HL et al. The selfish brain: competition for energy resources. *Prog Brain Res.* 2006;153:129–40.

Liu J et al. Reducing mitochondrial decay with mitochondrial nutrients to delay and treat cognitive dysfunction, Alzheimer's disease, and Parkinson's disease. *Nutr Neurosci.* 2005 Apr;8)2):67–89.

López-Lluch G et al. Mitochondrial biogenesis and healthy aging. *Exp Gerontol.* 2008 Sep;43(9):813–9.

Lau FC et al. Nutritional intervention in brain aging: reducing the effects of inflammation and oxidative stress. *Subcell Biochem.* 2007;42:299–318.

Hagiwara Y. *Green Barley Essence.* Keats Pub, Connecticut, 1985.

Schaffer S et al. Plant foods and brain aging: a critical appraisal. *Forum Nutr.* 2006;59:86–115.

Navarro A et al. Brain mitochondrial dysfunction in aging: conditions that improve survival, neurological performance and mitochondrial function. *Front Biosci.* 2007 Jan 1;12:1154–63.

Letenneur L et al. Flavonoid intake and cognitive decline over a 1-year period. *Am J Epidemiol.* 2007

Jun 15;165l12):1364–71.

Van der Schaft J et a.. The association between vitamin D and cognition: a systematic review. *Ageing Res Rev.* 2013 Sep;12(4):1013–23.

Zafra-Stone S et al. Berry anthocyanins as novel antioxidants in human health and disease prevention. *Mol Nutr Food Res.* 2007 Jun;51(6):675–83.

Krikorian R et al. Blueberry supplementation improves memory in older adults. *J Agric Food Chem.* 2010 Apr 14;58(7):3996–4000.

Shukitt-Hale B et al. Blueberry polyphenols attenuate kainic acid-induced decrements in cognition and alter inflammatory gene expression in rat hippocampus. *Nutr Neurosci.* 2008 Aug;11(4):172–82.

Zhu Y et al. Blueberry opposes beta-amyloid peptide-induced microglia. activation via inhibition of p44/42 mitogen-activation protein kinase. *Rejuvenation Res.* 2008 Oct;11(5):891–901.

Willis LM et al. Modulation of cognition and behavior in aged animals: role for antioxidant and essential fatty acid-rich plant foods. *Am J Clin Nutr.* 2009 May;89(5 :1602S–1502S.

Mazza G et al. Absorption of anthocyanins from blueberries and serum antioxidant status in human subjects. *J Agric Food Chem.* 2002 Dec 18;50(26 :7731–7.

Akbaraly NT et al. Plasma carotenoid levels and cognitive performance in an elderly population: results cf the EVA Study. *J Gerontol A Biol Sci Med Sci.* 2007 Mar;62(3):303–06.

Soni M et al. Vitamin D and cognitive function. *Scand J Clin Lab Invest Suppl.* 2012 Apr;243:79–82.

Kesse-Guyot E et al. French adults' cognitive performance after daily supplementation with antioxidant vitamins and minerals at nutritional doses: a post hoc analysis of the Supplementation in Vitamins and Mineral Antioxidants (SU.VI.MAX) trial. *Am J Clin Nutr.* 2011 Sep;94(3):892–9.

Holford P. *New Optimum Nutrition for the Mind*, 2nd edn. Basic Health Publications, London, 2009.

Davison KM et al. Vitamin and mineral intakes in

adults with mood disorders: comparisons to nutrition standards and associations with sociodemographic and clinical variables. *J Am Coll Nutr.* 2011 Dec;30(6):547–58.

Hickey S and Saul AW. *Vitamin C: the real story.* Basic Health Publications, Laguna Beach, CA, 2008.

Miller JW. Vitamin E and memory: is it vascular protection? *Nutr Rev.* 2000 Apr;58(4):109–11.

Joseph JA et al. Grape juice, berries, and walnuts affect brain ageing and behaviour. *J Nutr.* 2009 Sep;139(9):1813S–7S.

Ames BN. Low micronutrient intake may accelerate the degenerative diseases of aging through allocation of scarce micronutrients by triage. *Proc Natl Acad Sci.* 2006 Nov 21;103(47):17589–94.

Thomas, D. Chapter 2: Mental health and mineral depletion in *Nutrition and Mental Health: a handbook* by Watts, M (ed). Pavilion, Brighton, 2009.

Hong CH et al. Anemia and risk of dementia in older adults: findings from the Health ABC study. *Neurology.* 2013 Aug 6;81(6):528–33.

Chapter 5: Protein and communication in your brain

Young SN. Behavioural effects of dietary neurotransmitter precursors: basic and clinical aspects. *Neurosci Biobehav Rev.* 1996 Summer;20(2):313–23.

Wurtman RJ et al. Effects of the Diet on Brain Neurotransmitters. *Nut Rev.* 1974 July;32(7):193–200.

Cooper, JR et al. *The Biochemical Basis of Neuropharmacology*, 8th edn. Oxford University Press, New York, 2002.

Victoroff J. *Saving Your Brain: the revolutionary plan to boost brain power, improve memory, and protect yourself against aging and Alzheimer's.* Bantam Books, Milsons Point, 2002.

Osiecki H, Meeke F and Smith J. *The Encyclopedia of Clinical Nutrition: volume 1: the nervous system.* BioConcepts Publishing, Eagle Farm, 2004.

Braverman, ER. *The Healing Nutrients Within.* Basic Health Publications, California, 2003.

Healy D. *Let Them Eat Prozac: The unhealthy relationship between the pharmaceutical industry and depression.* NYU Press, New York, 2006.

Ioannidis JPA. Effectiveness of antidepressants: an evidence myth constructed from a thousand randomized trials? *Philos Ethics Humanit Med.* 2008 May 27;3:14.

Davis JM et al. Should we treat depression with drugs or psychological interventions? A reply to Ioannidis. *Philos Ethics Humanit Med.* 2011 May 10;6:8.

Fournier JC et al. Antidepressant drug effects and depression severity: a patient-level meta-analysis. *JAMA.* 2010 Jan 6;303(1):47–53.

Le Noury J et al. Restoring Study 329: efficacy and harms of paroxetine and imipramine in treatment of major depression in adolescence. *BMJ.* 2015;351:h4320.

Van de Weyer, C. *Changing Diets, Changing Minds: how food affects mental well being and behaviour.* Sustain Publication, London, 2006.

Feeding Minds: the impact of food on mental health. Mental Health Foundation, UK, 2006.

Geary A. *Food and Mood Handbook: find relief at last from depression, anxiety, PMS, cravings and mood swings.* Thorsons, London, 2001.

Pfeiffer, C and Holford, P. *Mental Illness: the nutrition connection.* ION Press, London, 1996.

Crawford, M. *Nutrition and Evolution.* Keats Pub, New Canaan, Connecticut, 1995.

Carper, J. *Your Miracle Brain.* Thorsons, London, 2000.

Campbell-McBride N. *Gut and Psychology Syndrome.* Medinform Publishing, Cambridge, 2010.

Sienkiewicz Sizer F, Piché LA, Whitney EN. *Nutrition: concepts and controversies*, 2nd edn, Nelson Education, Toronto, 2012.

Fernanda Laus M et al. Early postnatal

protein-calorie malnutrition and cognition: a review of human and animal studies. *Int J Env Res Pub Health*. 2011;8:590–612.

Wurtman RJ et al. Precursor control of neurotransmitter synthesis. *Pharmacol Rev*. 1981;32:315–35.

Wurtman RJ et al. Effects of diet on brain neurotransmitters. *Nutrition Reviews*. 1974;32(7):193–200.

Young SN. Behavioural effects of dietary neurotransmitter precursors: basic and clinical aspects. *Neurosci Biobehav Rev*. 1996 Summer;20(2):313–23.

Young SN. Amino Acids, Brain Metabolism, Mood and Behaviour in *Nutritional Neuroscience: Nutrition, Brain and Behaviour*. Edited by Lieberman HR, Kanarek RB, Prasad C. Taylor & Francis Group, Florida. 2005; chapters 9 and 10.

Jacobsen MB et al. Relation between food provocation and systemic immune activation in patients with food intolerance. *Lancet*. 2000 Jul 29;356(9227):400–1.

Young SN. Clinical Nutrition: 3. The fuzzy boundary between nutrition and psychopharmacology. *CMAJ*. Jan 2002;166(2): 205–9.

Chapter 6: Stable energy for your brain

Appleton N and Jacobs GN. *Suicide by Sugar: a startling look at our #1 national addiction*. Square One Pub, New York, 2009.

Fehm HL et al. The selfish brain: competition for energy resources. *Prog Brain Res*. 2006;153:129–40.

Singh Khalsa D and Stauth C. *The Mind Miracle*. Arrow Books, London, 1998.

Logan, AC. *The Brain Diet*. Cumberland House Publishing, Tennessee, 2007.

Gillespie D. *Sweet Poison: why sugar makes us fat*. Viking, Camberwell, 2008.

Gold PE. Glucose and age-related changes in memory. *Neurobiol Aging*. Dec 2005;26 Supple 1:60–4.

Pasinetti GM et al. Metabolic syndrome and the role of dietary lifestyles in Alzheimer's disease.

J Neurochem. 2008 Aug;106(4):1503–1514.

Benton D. The impact of the supply of glucose to the brain on mood and memory. *Nutr Rev*. 2001 Jan;59(1 Pt 2):S20–1

Chaplin K et al. Breakfast and snacks: associations with cognitive failures, minor injuries, accidents and stress. *Nutrients*. 2011 May;3(5):515–28.

Nilsson A et al. Effects on cognitive performance of modulating the postprandial blood glucose profile at breakfast. *Eur J Clin Nutr*. 2012 Sep;66(9):1039–43.

Smith D et al. Hypoglycemia unawareness and the brain. *Diabetologia*. 2002 Jul;45(7):949–58.

Emoto K. Dendrite remodeling in development and disease. *Dev Growth Differ*. 2011 Apr;53(3):277–286.

Leonard BE. Inflammation, depression and dementia: are they connected? *Neurochem Res*. 2007 Oct;32(10):1749–56.

Prasad C. *Nutritional Neuroscience: Nutrition, Brain and Behaviour* by Lieberman HR, Kanarek RB, Prasad C (eds). Taylor & Francis Group, Florida. 2005; chapters 5 and 6.

Stranahan AM et al. Diabetes impairs hippocampal function through glucocorticoid-mediated effects on new and mature neurons. *Nat Neurosci*. 2008 Mar;11(3):309–17.

Stranahan AM et al. Diet-induced insulin resistance impairs hippocampal synaptic plasticity and cognition in middle-aged rats. *Hippocampus*. 2008;18(11):1085–8.

Ward MA et al. The effect of body mass index on global brain volume in middle-aged adults: a cross sectional study. *BMC Neurol*. 2005 Dec 2;5:23.

Gosnell BA. Sucrose predicts rate of acquisition of cocaine self-administration. *Psychopharmacology*. 2000;149:286–92.

Schoenthaler SJ. The Los Angeles Probation Department Diet–Behaviour Program: an empirical analysis of six institutional settings. *Int J Biosocial Res*. 1983, 5(2):88–39.

Schoenthaler SJ. Northern California

Diet–Behaviour Program: an empirical examination of 3000 incarcerated juveniles in Stanislaus County Juvenile Hall. *Int J Biosocial Res*. 5(2):99–108.

Teff K et.al. Dietary fructose reduces circulating insulin and leptin, attenuates postprandial suppression of ghrelin, and increases triglycerides in women. *J Clin Endocronol Metab*. 2004 Jun;89(6):2963–72.

Gaby A. Adverse effects of dietary fructose. *Alternative Medicine Review*. 2005 10(4):294–306.

Moeller SM et al. The effects of high fructose syrup. *J Am Coll Nutr*. 2009 Dec;28(6):619–26.

Melcombe L. *Health Hazards of White Sugar*. Alive Books, Vancouver, 2000.

Neil K. Chapter 11: Blood Sugar Blues in *Nutrition and Mental Health: a handbook*. Watts, M (ed). Pavilion, Brighton, 2009.

Sharma RP et al. Effects of repeated doses of aspartame on serotonin and its metabolites in various regions of the mouse brain. *Food Chem Toxicol*. 1987 Aug;25(8):565–8.

Van Boxtel MP et al. The effects of habitual caffeine use on cognitive change: a longitudinal perspective. *Pharmacol Biochem Behav*. 2003 Jul;75(4):921–7.

Shilo L et al. The effects of coffee consumption on sleep and melatonin secretion. *Sleep Med*. 2002 May;3(3):271–3.

Uribarri J et al. Diet-derived advanced glycation end products are major contributors to the body's AGE pool and induce inflammation in healthy subjects. *Ann N Y Acad Sci*. 2006 Jun;1043:461–6.

Vlassara H. Advanced glycation in health and disease: role of the modern environment. *Ann N Y Acad Sci*. 2005 Jun;1043:452–60.

Uribarri J et al. Circulating glycotoxins and dietary advanced glycation end products: two links to inflammatory response, oxidative stress and aging. *Gerontol A Biol Sci Med Sci*. 2007 Apr;62(4):427–33.

Sembra RD et al. Does accumulation of advanced glycation end products contribute to the aging phenotype? *J Gerontol A Biol Sci Med Sci*. 2010 Sep;65(9):963–75.

Bittencourt Lda S et al. Guarana (Paullinia cupana Mart.) prevents beta-amyloid aggregation, generation of advanced glycation-end products (AGEs), and acrolein-induced cytotoxicity on human neuronal-like cells. *Phytother Res*. 2014 Nov;28(11):1615–24.

Chapter 7: The foundation fats for your brain

Allessandri JM et al. Polyunsaturated fatty acids in the central nervous system: evolution of concepts and nutritional implications throughout life. *Reprod Nutr Dev*. 2004 Nov–Dec; 44(6):509–38.

Sinn N. Oiling the brain: a review of randomized controlled trials of omega-3 fatty acids in psychopathology across the lifespan. *Nutrients*. 2010 Feb;2(2):128–70.

Hussain G et al. Fatting the brain: a brief of recent research. *Front Cell Neurosci*. 2013 Sep 9;7:144.

Blasbalg TL et al. Changes in consumption of omega-3 and omega-6 fatty acids in the United States during the 20th century. *Am J Clin Nutr*. 2011 May; 93(5): 950–62.

Chang CY et al. Essential fatty acids and human brain. *Acta Neurol Taiwan*. 2009 Dec; 18(4):231–41.

Cho HP et al. Cloning, expression, and nutritional regulation of the mammalian Delta-6 desaturase. *J Biol Chem*. 1999 Jan 1;274(1):471–7.

Carlson NR. *Physiology of Behavior*, 8th edn. University of Massachusetts, Amherst, Pearson Education, 2004.

Connor WE. Alpha-linolenic acid in health and disease. *Am J Clin Nutr*. 1999;69(5):827–8.

Cordain L et al. Origins and evolution of the Western diet: health implications of the 21st century. *Clin Nutr*. 2005;81(2):341–54.

Enig MG. *Know Your Fats: the complete primer for understanding the nutrition of fats, oils and cholesterol*. Bethesda Press, Silver Spring, 2000.

Erasmus U. *Fats That Heal, Fats That Kill*. Alive Books, Burnaby, 1993.

Heinrichs SC. Dietary omega-3 fatty acid

supplementation for optimizing neuronal structure and function. *Mol Nutr Food Res.* 2010 Apr;54(4):447–56.

Hibbeln JR. From homicide to happiness: a commentary on omega-3 fatty acids in human society. Cleave Award Lecture. *Nutr Health.* 2007;19(1–2):9–19.

Holman RT. The slow discovery of the importance of omega 3 essential fatty acids in human health. *J Nutr.* 1998 Feb;128(2 Suppl):427S–433S.

Kidd PM. Omega-3 DHA and EPA for cognition, behavior, and mood: clinical findings and structural-functional synergies with cell membrane phospholipids. *Altern Med Rev.* 2007 Sep;12(3):207–27.

McMillan Price and Davie J. *Star Foods.* ABC Books, Sydney, 2008.

Myers, DG. *Psychology*, 4th edn. Worth Publishers Inc, New York, 1995, p43.

Pan DA et al. Dietary lipid profile is a determinant of tissue phospholipid fatty acid composition and rate of weight gain in rats. *J Nutr.* 1993 Mar;123(3):512–9.

Peet M (ed). *Phospholipid Spectrum Disorder in Psychiatry.* Marius Press, Lancashire, 1999.

Roberts RO et al. Polyunsaturated fatty acids and reduced odds of MCI: the Mayo Clinic Study of Aging. *J Alzheimers Dis.* 2010;21(3):853–65.

Ros E. Health benefits of nut consumption. *Nutrients.* 2010;2(7):652–82.

Severus WE. Effects of omega-3 polyunsaturated fatty acids on depression. *Herz.* 2006 Dec;31(Suppl 3):69–74.

Simopoulos AP. Human requirement for N-3 polyunsaturated fatty acids. *Poult Sci.* 2000 Jul;79(7):961–70.

Thomas D. The mineral depletion of foods available to us as a nation (1940–2002): a review of the 6th edition of McCance and Widdowson. *Nutr and Health.* 2007;19(1–2):21–55.

Uauy R et al. Essential fatty acids in early life: structural and functional role. *Proc Nutr Soc.* 2000 Feb;59(1):3–15.

Weaver KL et al. Effect of dietary fatty acids on inflammatory gene expression in healthy humans. *J Biol Chem.* 2009 Jun 5;284(23):15400–7.

Wahrburg U. What are the health effects of fat? *Eur J Nutr.* 2004 Mar;43(Suppl 1) I/6–11.

Layé S. What do you eat? Dietary omega 3 can help to slow the aging process. *Brain Behav Immun.* 2013 Feb;28:14–5.

Amarasiri WA et al. Coconut fats. *Ceylon Med J.* 2006 Jun; 51(2): 47–51.

Alexander JC. Chemical and biological properties related to toxicity of heated fats. *J Toxicol Environ Health.* 1981 Jan; 7(1): 125–38.

Bird RP et al. Cytotoxicity of thermally oxidized fats. *In Vitro.* 1981 May; 17(5): 397–404.

Kanner J. Dietary advanced lipid oxidation end products are risk factors to human health. *Mol Nutr Food Res.* 2007 Sep;51(9):1094–101.

Murray S et al. Chewing the fat on trans fats. *Can Med Assoc J.* 8 Nov 2005;173(10):1158–9.

Prabhu HR. Lipid peroxidation in culinary oils subjected to thermal stress. *Indian J Clin Biochem.* 2000 Aug;15(1):1–5.

Qu YH et al. Genotoxicity of heated cooking oil vapors. *Mutation Res.* 1992 Dec;298(2):105–11.

Mozaffarian D et al. Fish intake, contaminants, and human health: evaluating the risks and the benefits. *JAMA.* 2006 Oct 18;296(15):1385–99.

Spiteller G. The relation of lipid per oxidation processes with atherogenesis: a new theory on atherogenesis. *Mol Nutr Food Res.* 2005 Nov;49(11):999–1013.

Williams MJ et al. Impaired endothelial function following meal rich in used cooking fat. *J Am Collins Cardiol.* 1999 Mar 15;33(4):1050–5.

Wilson B. *Swindled: the dark history of food fraud, from poisoned candy to counterfeit coffee.* Princeton University Press, New Jersey, 2008.

Wu TH et al. Salmon by-product storage and oil extraction. *Food Chemistry.* April 2008;111:868–71.

Cleland LG et al. Fish oil: what the prescriber needs to know. *Arthritis Res Ther.* 2006; 8(1):202.

Goldberg RJ et al. A meta-analysis of the analgesic effects of omega-3 polyunsaturated fatty acid supplementation for inflammatory joint pain. *Pain.* May 2007;129(1–2):210–23.

Goyens PL et al. Conversion of alpha-linolenic acid in humans is influenced by the absolute amounts of alpha-linolenic acid and linoleic acid in the diet and not by their ratio. *Am J Clin Nutr.* 2006 Jul;84(1):44–53.

Umhau JC et al. Imaging incorporation of circulating docosahexaenoic acid into the human brain using positron emission tomography. *J Lipid Res.* 2009 Jul;50(7):1259–68.

Williams CM et al. Long-chain n-3 PUFA: plant v. marine sources. *Proc Nutr Soc.* 2006 Feb;65(1):42–50.

Yehuda S et al. Essential fatty acids are mediators of brain biochemistry and cognitive functions. *J Neurosci Res.* 1999 Jun 15;56(6):565–70.

Zamaria N. Alteration of polyunsaturated fatty acid status and metabolism in health and disease. *Reprod Nutr Dev.* May–Jun 2004;44(3):273–82.

Zhang W et al. Omega-3 polyunsaturated fatty acids in the brain: metabolism and neuroprotection. *Front Bioscience.* 2011 Jun 1;17:2653–70.

Alumudena Sánchez-Villegas et al. Dietary fat intake and the risk of depression: the SUN Project. *PLoS One.* 2011 Jan 26:6(1):e16268.

Peet M. Essential fatty acids: theoretical aspects and treatment implications for schizophrenia and depression. *Advances in Psychiatric Treatment.* 2002;8:223–9.

Perica MM et al. Essential fatty acids and psychiatric disorders. *Nutr Clin Pract.* 2011 Aug;26(4):409–25.

Cakiner-Egilmez T. Omega 3 fatty acids and the eye. *Insight.* 2008 Oct–Dec;33(4):20–5; quiz 26–7.

Dullemeijer C et al. Plasma very long-chain N-3 polyunsaturated fatty acids and age-related hearing loss in older adults. *J Nutr Health Aging.* 2010;14(5):347–51.

Miner JL et al. Conjugated linoleic acid (CLA), body fat, and apoptosis. *Obes Res.* 2001 Feb;9(2):129–34.

Shelton RC and Miller SH. Eating ourselves to death and despair: the contribution of adiposity and inflammation to depression. *Prog Neurobiol.* 2010 August;91(4):275–99.

Basu S et al. Conjugated linoleic acid induces lipid peroxidation in men with abdominal obesity. *Clin Sci (Lond).* 2000 Dec;99(6):511–6.

Medina EA et al. Conjugated linoleic acid supplementation in humans: effects on circulating leptin concentrations and appetite. *Lipids.* 2000 Jul;35(7):783–8.

Tassoni D et al. The role of eicosanoids in the brain. *Asia Pac J Clin Nutr.* 2008;17 (Suppl 1):220–8.

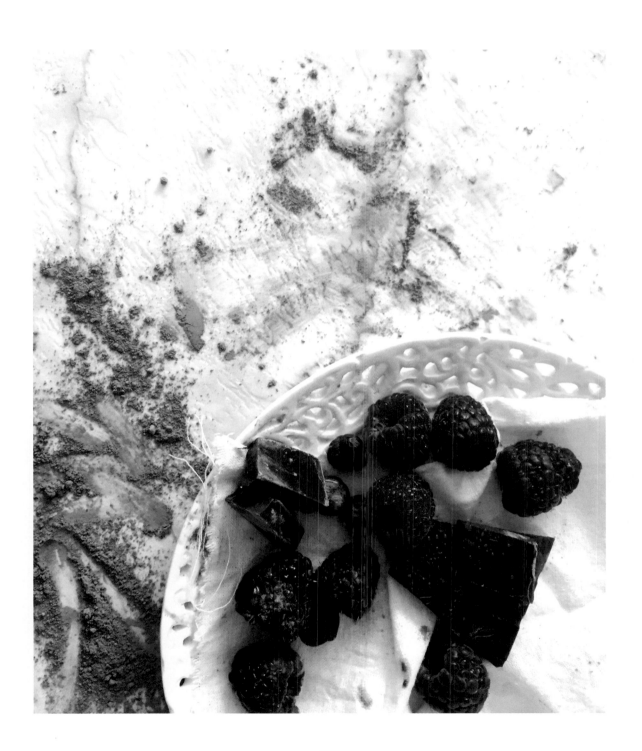

General index

General index

General index

Recipe index